Deep Sleep with Hypnosis for Women

Say Bye-Bye to Anxiety, Insomnia Struggle and Bad Habits Before Bed | Find out Mind-Body Relaxation with Ocean Visualization to Fall Asleep Quickly and Sleep Well

Jackie Parks

Table of Contents

Introduction 3

Chapter 1   Induction 8

Chapter 2   Before Bed Hypnosis 13

Chapter 3   Mind-Body Relaxation to Decrease Stress and Anxiety 17

Chapter 4   Sleep Hypnosis Scripts 33

Chapter 5   Guided Meditation: 30 Minute Deep Sleep Hypnosis for Better Sleep, Stress Relief, & Relaxation   38

Chapter 6   Better Sleep Habits 43

Chapter 7   Deep Sleep Hypnosis - Sleepy Ocean Visualization 46

Chapter 8	Deep Sleep Techniques	51
Chapter 9	Sleep Meditation	58
Chapter 10	Meditation for Stress Relief	61
Chapter 11	Affirmation	67
Chapter 12	Understanding Hypnosis - History, Benefits, and Uses	71
Chapter 13	The First Steps to Ending the Insomnia Struggle	78
Conclusion		84

Introduction

We in general consider sleep when our mind and body shut down. Instead sleep is a functioning period wherein a great deal of significant handling, reclamation, and reinforcing happens. Precisely how this occurs and why is still fairly a secret. In any case, we do know the importance of benefits of sleep, and the reasons we need it for ideal well-being and prosperity.

One of the indispensable jobs of sleep is to enable us to cement and combine memories which we gather during the day. As we approach our day, our mind takes in a lot of data. Instead of being straightforwardly logged and recorded, these actualities and encounters first should be handled and put away; and a considerable lot of these means occur while we sleep.

Medium-term, odds and ends of data are moved from progressively provisional, transient memory to more grounded, long haul memory—a procedure called "solidification." Researchers have demonstrated that after individuals rest, they are able to hold more information and perform better on memory errands. Our bodies require bedtimes to reestablish and revive, to develop muscle, fix tissue, and combine hormones. Yet we ignore sleep for other things. The National Sleep Foundation gives recommendations on how much sleep people should get at each age:

Age Group	Recommended sleep duration per day
Newborns	14–17 hours
Infants	12–15 hours
Toddlers	11–14 hours
Preschoolers	10–13 hours
School Age	9–11 hours
Teen	8–10 hours
Young Adults and Adults	7–9 hours
Older Adults	7–8 hours

Proper rest is basic for everybody, since us as a whole need to hold information and learn aptitudes to sail through everyday life. Be that as it may, this is likely piece of the reason youngsters—who procure language, social, and engine abilities at a stunning pace all through their advancement—need more rest than grown-ups. While grown-ups need at least 8 hours of sleep for each night, one-year-olds need 17 hours, school age youngsters somewhere in the range of 9 to 11, and adolescents somewhere in the range of 8 and 10. During these basic times of development and learning, young individuals need a substantial portion of sleep for ideal advancement and readiness.

Unfortunately, an individual cannot simply amass lack of sleep and after that log numerous long periods of rest to compensate for it. The best rest propensities are steady, solid schedules that permit us all, paying little heed to our age, to meet our sleep needs each night, and keep over life's difficulties consistently.

According to the US Department of Health about 35% of the adults in United States sleeps less than 7 hours a day. Meanwhile sleep deprivation can have severe consequences on our health and lifestyle: adults who were short sleepers were more likely to report chronic health problems, obesity and physical inactivity compared to people who got enough sleep.

Although how long you sleep each day is very important, healthy sleep has more to do with quality of rest than quantity of hours. A good sleep quality is essential and contribute to your health and well-being.

Inadequate sleep affects both how we feel and how we function. Short-term effects can include sleepiness or drowsiness, reduced alertness, irritability, attention and reaction problems, poor motor skills. Regularly sleeping less than seven hours increases the risk of developing diabetes, heart disease, mood disorders, unhealthy eating habits that can lead to other chronic illnesses. Chronic sleep problems can link to depression, anxiety, and mental distress.

What Keeps People Up at Night?

At some random time, most of the individuals are experiencing issues related to peaceful resting. Difficulty in sleeping, non-getting enough rest, constantly worrying about insomnia, and the build-up of stress and frustration as a result is what has seeped into the modern lifestyle. Practically everybody encounters times of restlessness sooner or later in their life.

Many people lament they experience sleep problems. It is a term that describes several different sleep issues, including:

- Not getting enough sleep (sleep deprivation or insufficient sleep).
- Not sleeping well.
- Not spending enough time in certain stages of sleep.
- Having a sleep disorder (such as insomnia, sleep apnea, narcolepsy and others).

There are many possible reasons for sleeping difficulties, including lifestyle, sleeping habits, and medical conditions. Generally, decreased rest stem from an overactive routine, from a stress feeling, or even from a physical condition. Similarly, emotional wellness issues can prompt poor rest. A sleeping disorder can be activated or propagated by your practices and erratic sleep pattern. Irregular ways of life and rest propensities can give rise to a sleeping disorder (with no fundamental mental or medical issue).

There are some other reasons which keep people up at night. Too warm room temperature, not dark enough room, external sounds - all of that can disturb you. The stress of job, the addiction to be online all the time on mobile phones, tablets and laptops, relationship problems, financial issues, irregular food habits, drinking caffeine or smoking before bedtime, and many more are the reasons why people find it hard to get a deep restoring sleep. Overthinking, clockwatching, getting up to watch TV until one feels sleepy, talking on phones - everything contributes to a bad sleep pattern.

Nowadays, many people attend gym after work; sadly, it doesn't help to sleeping properly. Also, weekend parties where drinking alcohol too late has become a norm, mess up with the regular sleep cycle. If not addressed on time it will snowball into a bigger problem resulting in physical and psychological problems.

One of the biggest contributors of sleeplessness is the technology, keeping aside the health issues and everyday problems. Our mobile phones, tablets, PCs and other electronic devices have turned out to be such a gigantic piece of our day by day experience that it's regularly difficult to put them down—even at sleep time. Keeping your smartphone or other devices on your end table may not appear to be a major deal, yet innovation influences your rest in a larger number of ways than you understand.

Wanting to sleep but not getting to sleep is the cycle which can be ceaseless. The realization about sleeplessness doesn't help either. The more time is spent on worrying about it, the farther goes its solution. Sadly, our fast-paced lifestyle is full of roadblocks, so it is very important to pause and contemplate on our surroundings and actions which lead us to becoming restless, thus contributing to our poor sleep.

A healthy mind is crucial to healthy functioning of your body. Our bodies are biological machines which need to rest at appropriate intervals. Effective techniques are to be followed to code and train our mind in such a way that sleep comes naturally, without minimal efforts. Worrying about lack of sleep is going to drive it away further. What is needed is to seek solutions and keeping your mind clear of stressful energy which hinders peaceful rest.

Why Practice Sleep Meditation?

Meditation is a simple process of relaxing the mind. The sleep meditation practice could become a calming and relaxing ritual, that will help you to sleep better all night. It can also help you to let go the worries of the day, to combat weakness and a sleep disorders.

Meditation – the act of purposefully calming or centering the mind – makes physiological changes that are like those that occur in your body during the early periods of rest. Your heartbeat eases back, circulatory strain drops, and stress hormones decline. Meditation is fit for upgrading your focus, diminishing stress, overseeing physical and mental pain, bringing down your high blood pressure and, in addition to other things – improve your sleep quality.

Day by day meditation practice will help you to loosen up your body and to relax yourself faster and easier. You will be able to fall asleep instantly, overcome insomnia, reduce anxiety and stress, sleep smarter and wake up energized.

Many sleep-related difficulties may be solved trying meditation. Sleep meditation helps create the inner conditions needed for a truly restful night. The deep breathing and relaxation techniques are useful to improve sleep quality, increase sleep time, and make it easier to fall (and stay) asleep. These are some benefits of meditation and relaxation practices:

- Meditation is safe. It can be a great medication-free way to treat sleep disorders. Also, there are no associated risks or side effects to trying meditation.

- Practicing meditation before sleep leads to relaxation, happiness and optimism. Happiness hormones are triggered as you meditate, which leaves you in a good mood when you wake up. It also improves insomnia symptoms, stress and fatigue.

- Meditation can help to improve the quality and efficiency of sleep, how quickly you fall asleep, and how long you can stay awake during the day.

- Meditation is easy. It is an accessible, budget-friendly practice that everyone can try.

- Meditation can be used with other treatments.

- Meditation has multiple health benefits. It can not only improve your sleep quality, but it may also help reduce blood pressure and ease pain, anxiety, and depression. Improved sleep also affects our immune systems, wellbeing and health, encourages better eating habits and weight management.

Taking a cue from sleep meditation and similar practices, here is a guide to peaceful sleeping which intends to put your sleeping pattern on the right track. From effective breathing and relaxation techniques to diet tips, we have garnered essential information for your overall well-being. Drifting into a peaceful slumber would become an easier task with the information in this book. Making you a smart sleeper is what you will be getting here. Because rest is important, and so are you.

Chapter 1   Induction

At this point in the audio, I invite you to make yourself as comfortable as possible in your bed. Please have all the light's turned off and distractions put away. You have already put in a full, hard day of work. Think of sleeping sound and comfortable through the night as a reward for working so hard.

How was your day today?

Were you productive?

How did you feel?

I want you to think about these questions as you settle further into the bed. Gently tuck yourself under the cover, and we will begin our journey. Ready?

Inhale deeply. Hold onto that breath for a moment, and then let it go. To begin, I am going to lead you through an induction script for self-hypnosis. By allowing yourself to slip into this state of mind, it will help you let go of any stress you may be holding onto, even if it is in your subconscious. I am going to help you tap into these emotions so you can let them go and sleep like you never have before.

All of us are stressed. Honestly, who can sleep when they are worried? In this state of mind, you probably feel too alert to even think about sleeping. When you are stressed, the adrenal glands in your body release adrenaline and cortisol. Both of these hormones keep you awake and stop you from falling asleep.

In the audio to follow, we will go over letting go of your worries, even if it is just for the night. You are in a safe place right now. Anything you need to get done can wait until tomorrow. It is important you take this time for yourself. We all need a break from our responsibilities at some point or another. I invite you now to take another deep breath so we can focus on what is important right now; sleep.

To start, I would like you to close your eyes gently. As you do this, wiggle slightly until your body feels comfortable in your bed. When you find your most comfortable position, it is time to begin breathing.

As you focus on your breath, remind yourself to breathe slow and deep. Feel as the air fills your lungs and release it in a comfortable way. Feel as your body relaxes further under the sheets. You begin to feel a warm glow, wrapping your whole body in a comfortable blanket.

Before you let go into a deep hypnotic state, listen carefully to the words I am saying at this moment.

Everything is going to happen automatically.

At this moment, there is nothing you need to focus on. You will have no control over what happens next in our session. But you are okay with that. At this moment, you are warm and safe. You are preparing your body for a full night's rest and letting go of any thoughts you may have. There is no need to think of the future or the past. The only thing that matters right now is your comfort, your breath, and the incredible sleep you are about to experience.

Now, feel as the muscles around your eyes begin to relax. I invite you to continue breathing deeply and bring your attention to your eyes. They are beginning to feel heavy and relaxed. Your eyes worked hard for you today. They watched as you worked, they kept you safe as you walked around, and they showed other people you were paying attention to them as you spoke. Thank your eyes at this moment and allow them to rest for the night so they will be prepared for tomorrow.

Your breath is coming easy and free now. Soon, you will enter a hypnotic trance with no effort. This trance will be deep, peaceful, and safe. There is nothing for your conscious mind to do at this moment. There are no activities you need to complete. Allow for your subconscious mind to take over and do the work for you.

This trance will come automatically. Soon, you will feel like you are dreaming. Allow yourself to relax and give in to my voice. All you need to focus on is my voice.

You are doing wonderfully. Without noticing, you have already changed your rate of breath. You are breathing easy and free. There is no thought involved. Your body knows exactly what you need to do, and you can relax further into your subconscious mind.

Now, you are beginning to show signs of drifting off into this peaceful hypnotic trance. I invite you to enjoy the sensations as your subconscious mind takes over and listens to the words I am speaking to you. It is slowly becoming less important for you to listen to me. Your subconscious listens, even as I begin to whisper.

You are drifting further and further away. You are becoming more relaxed and more comfortable. At this moment, nothing is bothering you. Your inner mind is listening to me, and you are beginning to realize that you don't care about slipping into a deep trance.

This peaceful state allows you to be comfortable and relaxed. Being hypnotized is pleasant and enjoyable. This is beginning to feel natural for you. Each time I hypnotize you, it becomes more enjoyable than the time before.

You will enjoy these sensations. You are comfortable. You are peaceful. You are completely calm.

As we progress through the relaxing exercises, you will learn something new about yourself. You are working gently to develop your own sleep techniques without even knowing you are developing them in the first place.

On the count of three, you are going to slip completely into your subconscious state. When I say the number three, your brain is going to take over, and you will find yourself in the forest. This forest is peaceful, calm, and serene. It is safe and comfortable, much like your bed at this moment. Take a deep breath in and exhale…you are ready for your journey.

One…

Two…

Three…

Welcome to the peaceful forest.

Before we begin, I want you to inhale deeply and hold onto the breath for three seconds. Once you have held the breath for three seconds, exhale slowly. You can breathe on my count. Ready?

Breathe in…two…three…four…hold…two…three…four…exhale…two…three…four.

Wonderful. You are doing a fantastic job. Let's do that a few more times.

Breathe in…two…three…four…hold…two…three…four…exhale…two…three…four.

Breathe in…two…three…four…hold…two…three…four…exhale…two…three…four

Breathe in…two…three…four…hold…two…three…four…exhale…two…three…four

As you inhale, try to bring more oxygen into your body with nice, deep breaths. As you exhale, feel as your body relaxes more and more into the bed. Breathing comes easy and free for you. As you continue to focus on your breath, you are becoming more peaceful and calmer without even realizing it.

As we continue, you do not care how relaxed you are. You are happy in the state of mind. You do not have a care in the world. Your subconscious mind is always aware of the words I am saying to you. As we go along, it is becoming less important for you to listen to my voice.

Your inner mind is receiving everything I tell you. Your conscious mind is relaxed and peaceful. As you find your own peace of mind, we will begin to explore this forest you have found yourself in, together.

Now, I want you to imagine you are laying near a stream in this beautiful and peaceful forest. It is a sunny, warm summer day. As you lay comfortably in the grass beside this stream, you feel a warm breeze, gently moving through your hair. Inhale deep and experience how fresh and clean this air is. Inhale again and exhale. Listen carefully as the stream flows beside you. A quiet whoosh noise, filling your ears and relaxing you even further.

It is becoming less and less important for you to listen to me. Your subconscious mind takes hold and listens to everything I am saying. All you need to do is enjoy the beautiful nature around you. The sunlight shines through the trees and kisses your skin gently. The birds begin to sing a happy tune. You smile, feeling yourself become one with nature.

Each time you exhale, I want to imagine your whole body relaxing more. You are becoming more at ease. As you do this, I want you to begin to use your imagination. You are lying on the grass. It is located in a green meadow with the sun shining down on you. The sun is not hot, but a comfortable warm.

Imagine that there are beautiful flowers blooming everywhere around you. Watch as the flowers move gently in the breeze. Their scents waft toward your nose as you inhale deeply and exhale.

When you are ready, I want you to imagine that you begin to stand up. As you do this, you look over your left shoulder gently, and you see a mountain near the edge of the beautiful meadow. You decide that you would like to take a trip up to the top of the mountain to see this beautiful view from a different angle.

As you begin to walk, you follow the stream. Imagine gently bending over and placing your hand not the cool, rushing water. As you look upon the water, imagine how clean and cool this water is. The stream flows gently across your fingers and it relaxes you.

When you are ready, we will head toward the mountain again. As you grow closer to the mountain, the birds begin to chirp. Inhale deep and imagine how the pine trees smell around you. Soon, you begin to climb the mountain at a comfortable pace.

You are enjoying the trip. It is wonderful to be outside with this beautiful nature, taking in all the sights and sounds. Now, you are already halfway up the mountain. The meadow grows smaller as you climb higher, but you are not afraid. The scene is beautiful from up here, and you are happy at this moment.

As you reach the top, take a deep breath and give yourself a pat on the back for your accomplishment. Take a look down on the meadow and see how small the trees look.

The breeze is blowing your hair around gently, and the sun continues to shine down on the top of your head. Imagine that you are taking a seat at the very top of the mountain. You close your eyes in your mind's eye and take a few moments to appreciate this nature. You wish you could always be this relaxed.

When you take your life into your own hands, you will be able to. This is why we are here. Of course, you may be here because you want to sleep, but you can't do that truly unless you learn how to let go of your stress. Through guided meditation and exercises within this audio, you will learn how to become a better version of yourself. I am here to help you every step of the way.

Soon, we will work on deepening your trance. You are beginning to relax further into the meditation and are opening your heart and soul to the practice. Remember that you are safe, and you are happy to be here.

Chapter 2   Before Bed Hypnosis

In order for us to dive deeper into your subconscious, I will need you to relax as much as you can. In the following few minutes, we are going to try a muscle relaxation exercise. As I mention an area, I invite you to focus on the area, so you can tense and relax it. When I tell you to tense an area, this should not cause you any pain whatsoever. If at any point you feel discomfort, please stop or try to ease up on tensing the area.

When you are ready, take a deep breath. Inhale…exhale…and we will begin.

We are first going to start with your neck and your shoulders.

To start, please try to raise your shoulders up toward your ears. As you do this, you will feel the muscles in your neck and shoulders begin to tighten. Feel the tension, where it builds, and then release. Allow your shoulders to drop to their normal position. Your shoulders and neck should feel comfortable. If not, try this again until you feel the muscles release and relax.

Remember to breathe through this process. Inhale…and exhale. Good.

Now, we will move onto your hands.

I want you to squeeze both hands into fists. Your hands are in very tight balls. You can try to pretend that you are squeezing a rubber ball. Hold this ball in your hands and feel as the tension begins to build first in your hands, and gently moves up your forearms.

When you feel the pressure, release your hands. Gently shake them and get rid of any tension. How do your hands feel now? They should feel much more relaxed.

With your neck and hands relaxed, let us draw your attention to your forehead. Our faces do a lot of activity for us through the day. Our facial expressions allow us to tell people when we are happy, sad, or stressed. I want you to raise your eyebrows. Feel as the muscles in your forehead begin to tighten and hold that position. Now, try to lower your eyebrows and tighten your eyes. Hold this tight for a few moments and then release.

Notice now how relaxed and smooth your forehead feels now that you have released the tension. Your eyelids are gently resting over your eyes, and you feel comfortable again. When you are ready, inhale…exhale…now move your focus to your jaw.

If you can, tightly close your mouth. Feel how tight your jaw feels as you clamp it closed. Your lips are tense across your teeth, and the tension builds in your jaw. Take a moment to note how this feels, and then relax your jaw. Allow your mouth to fall relaxed and loose. Release all tension and feel how wonderful and light your head feels.

To complete your relaxation, we will now practice deep breathing. Deep breathing is an excellent practice as it can help cure any stress or anxiety you may be feeling at any given moment. As you breathe, you remind your body that this is a fundament to your survival. Any time we are stressed, you may not notice, but our breathing patterns change. By doing this, it is your body's attempt to survive physical activity.

While helpful in actual dangerous situations, it won't help you if you are anxious over something that is isn't dangerous to you immediately. When our breathing becomes rapid, it also becomes shallow. Short, shallow breaths may make you feel like you are unable to catch your breath. This is because you are not breathing properly.

When we do not breathe properly, your lungs fill with stale, old air. This is not helpful as new air is unable to enter. In this sense, you need oxygen to fill yourself with positive energy. Proper breathing techniques will help you in multiple ways from relaxing to letting go of stress. When you learn to breathe the right way, you can stop the negative cycle and gain the ability to calm your body under stressful circumstances.

If you find yourself breathing too quickly, it could cause tingling, numbness, or even lightheadedness. The cure here is to learn how to slow down your breathing. Bring your focus on keeping your breath deep and full.

Now, I am going to go through a breathing exercise with you. Before we begin, I want you to take careful note of how you are breathing right now. Are your lungs full? Do you feel like you have old air stuck in there? Are your breaths quick or long?

When you are ready, I want you to inhale slowly and count to four…We will pause and count to three…and then exhale to the count of five. Ready?

Wonderful. Let us try it a few more times. Truly try to focus on each step of your breath. Trust the natural rhythm of your breathing to help relieve any anxiety or stress you may be holding onto.

With your breath in mind, it is now time to give in completely to relaxation. It is time to assure your body and mind are both set for the session. Now, I want you to repeat after me, and then we will begin.

I am gently going into a state of total relaxation

(Pause)

At this moment, my body and mind are both relaxing.

(Pause)

I am going deeper and deeper. I am relaxing deeper and deeper.

(Pause)

Every muscle in my body is relaxing. I feel peaceful. Everything around me is quiet.

(Pause)

Wonderful. Now, I am going to count from the number one to the number ten. When I reach ten, your whole body will be relaxed. You will be safe and completely calm in your mind and in your soul. When you are ready, take a deep breath, exhale, and we will begin.

One…feel as all of the muscles in your face begin to relax. You are releasing the tension from your forehead. The muscles around your eyes soften. You allow your jaw to go slack. Your face was active all day long. At this moment, it is time to give your face a rest.

Two…the muscles in your neck begin to melt. They are loosening and relaxing. Your neck worked all day to keep your head on straight. Feel as the muscles relax and melt into your pillow and bed. They can finally rest up for another day.

Three…Feel as your shoulders relax further into the bed. If there is any tension in them, shake them out gently and allow them to fall away from your ears. Many of us hold our shoulders scrunched up through the day. We do it subconsciously when we are scared, stressed, or even just cold. Allow your shoulders to relax completely and feel them fall peacefully onto the bed without a care in the world.

Four…Gently bring your focus to your hands. They are finally done for the day. They held your food for you, typed away on the computer, and held your loved one. Now, they are free of any responsibility. Give them a quick flex and relax your hands. Allow your fingers to fall away from your fists and allow them to rest wherever they are at this moment.

Five…as the rest of your body begins to rest, feel as your chest muscles relax. They follow suit from your neck and your shoulders. Focus on the lungs inside of your chest. Breathing is coming easily and naturally. Each time you breathe, you feel yourself relax further into your meditation. Peacefully, thank your lungs for doing such a wonderful job to support you.

Six…imagine the muscles in your back begin to loosen. As you lay in bed, they are finally able to relax. They worked hard all day to keep you upright and supported you when you needed them most. Now, they can relax and enjoy a good night's rest. Feel as the muscles in your back and lower back let go of any final tension.

Seven…now, the muscles in your stomach are relaxing. If you were stressed today, you might have felt a lot of tension in your stomach. This is why we use the expressions "butterflies in my stomach" or "I felt sick to my stomach." There are many connections between our psyche and our stomachs. At this moment, you have no worries. Your stomach can relax and rest for the night.

Eight…feel the muscles of your buttock begin to relax. This is a location many of us don't spend a lot of time thinking about. Feel as the muscles loosen and relax. Your buttock sinks deeper into the bed, and you feel yourself becoming even more comfortable as your body gets ready for a full night's rest.

Nine…the top of your thighs is relaxing. Your legs do so much work through the day. They allow you to walk from place to place and support you. Gently release any tension that may be built up in your legs and picture them sinking deeper and more comfortable into the bed.

Ten…finally, feel like the muscles in your lower legs relax. Your feet let go of all tension, and you find yourself completely comfortable. There is not a single place in your body holding onto tension. You feel comfortable, safe, and at peace.

Now, you are in a state of total and deep relaxation. From the top of your head to the tip of your toes, you are totally relaxed.

You are feeling better and better. You are ready to focus on sleep at the count of three.

One…

Two…

Three…

Chapter 3   Mind-Body Relaxation to Decrease Stress and Anxiety

The purpose of this mind-body relaxation meditation is to get rid of fear and anxiety. This guided meditation session will take you deep inside your mind. You will be able to get rid of your fears and anxieties. You will get a chance to face them and defeat them.

This guided meditation is very helpful in relieving stress and anxiety. It helps you in sleeping better and provide complete physical, mental, and emotional relief. You can practice it anytime you like.

Take your position at the place of your meditation

Take your seat

Sit in a completely relaxed manner

Don't do anything immediately

Ground yourself first

Just sit completely relaxed for a few minutes

If something important comes to your mind write it down

If there is something that is bothering you, write it down

Get into a comfortable position

Keep your back straight

Ensure that your shoulders are also straight

Your back and neck should be in a straight line

Now, close your eyes

Lean slightly forward and then backward

Lean-to your left side and then to your right

Now, bring yourself to the center and find the best and most comfortable position

Feel your head positioned on your neck

Raise your chin slightly upwards

This will help you in placing your focus between your eyebrows

Try to feel your whole body

Notice if there is tension anywhere

If you feel any part tense, release the tension

Adjust your body to release the pressure

This meditation will help you in relaxing your body and mind

You will let go of all your stress and anxiety

Throughout the meditation session

You will breathe in through your nose slowly

Hold your breath for a few seconds

Breathe out through your mouth making a "Haaaaa" sound

It might look like you are testing your breath

This process helps in taking out all the spent air from your body

It takes away the stress and anxiety

Breathe in slowly through your nostrils

Let it fill your abdomen

Let it light your body

Hold the breath for a few seconds

Now exhale with the 'Haaaa'

Repeat the process 5 times

Breathe in slowly through your nostrils

Let it fill your abdomen

Let it light your body

Hold the breath for a few seconds

Exhale with the 'Haaaa'

Breathe in slowly through your nostrils

Let it fill your abdomen

Let it light your body

Hold the breath for a few seconds

Exhale with the 'Haaaa'

Breathe in slowly through your nostrils

Let it fill your abdomen

Let it light your body

Hold the breath for a few seconds

Exhale with the 'Haaaa'

Breathe in slowly through your nostrils

Let it fill your abdomen

Let it light your body

Hold the breath for a few seconds

Exhale with the 'Haaaa'

Breathe in slowly through your nostrils

Let it fill your abdomen

Let it light your body

Hold the breath for a few seconds

Exhale with the 'Haaaa'

You are feeling much relaxed and composed now

There is no stress and anxiety in the body

You are feeling comfortable

You are feeling calm

If there were thoughts bothering you?

They have disappeared now

It is time to relax your breathing

There is no rush now

There is no fear now

You can bring your breathing to normal

Breathe in slowly

Hold the breath

Exhale through your mouth

Don't count

Don't bother

Let your body find its breathing rhythm

Let's not bother about it

Shift your focus between your eyes

Keep your eyes comfortably closed

Do not squint your eyes

Simply try to see the light between your eyebrows

Somewhere in the center of your forehead

You might see the white fog a bit above the center of your nose bridge

Enter this fog

There is something beyond this fog

It looks very peaceful

You should explore it

There is no need to be anxious

Enter the fog

The fog is not very dense

On the other side of the fog, there is a green pasture

It's a lush green grassland

It's so green that even a single yellow blade of grass can be spotted

You haven't seen such lush green pasture in years

It is mesmerizing

It is so soothing to the eyes

You are loving the scenery

You wanted to visit such a place for so long

It is like a dream come true

Look all around yourself

There are some sheep grazing the green grass

They are so white as if wearing snowflakes

Not even a single sheep has patches of color

Looks like they have been painted

But they are real

They are not inanimate

They are moving

Making noise

At the other side, there are some kids

They are playing

The kids are trying to throw stones as far as possible

It is such an amusing game

They are small kids

Not very powerful

They can't throw the stones very far

Their stones fall very near

You like this game

But you don't want to disturb the kids

You look at the other side

There is a valley

Very deep

Very steep

It looks like you are at the edge of a cliff

You find some stones lying there

You want to play the same game

You want to test your throwing arm

You used to be really good at it

There is no harm in trying again

There is no one looking at it

There is nothing to be ashamed of

You pick up a pebble

It looks small

But it is heavy

Just like your fears and anxieties

They are also small and insignificant in size

But they keep you anxious

They keep you worried

You just can't seem to stop thinking about them

It is a good time to get rid of them

No one is here to notice you

Pick up each stone and fling it hard

Throw it from here

It cannot return

You can get rid of all your fears and anxieties here

No one will notice you

You will come out of here fearless

You will not have these anxieties

You will be able to get rid of them

Pick up a stone

Think of it as some generalized fear

Begin with small things that worry you

Pick anyone

Now throw it hard

It feels good

You are feeling relieved

This is an amazing feeling

You can get rid of all your fears and anxieties here

You have all the time and opportunity here

Let's try another one

Pick any of your bigger worries

Look at it fearlessly

Face it

It can't scare you anymore

You can throw it away at any moment

Now get rid of it

Isn't it an exhilarating feeling?

You have started enjoying the process now

Let's try a bigger one

Pick the things that make you anxious

Pick the things that have been making you insecure

The things that scare you the most

Weigh it in your hands

It didn't weigh that much after all

Yet, you remain scared of it

Face it now

Look at it for the last time

It should know that you are victorious now

You have conquered it

Now, let's try something that makes you really restless

Don't be afraid

There's nothing that they can do

You are in complete control

You are not afraid of anything now

You have taken the matters in your own hands now

Pick it up

Face it

Call out its name loudly

Louder

Even louder so that you can hear it

Louder so that even the kids can hear you

There is no shame in facing your fears

You are challenging them now

You are one step away from conquering them all

Fling it forward into the deep abyss

It's gone now

Gone forever

You have won

You have become victorious over your fears

You are feeling great

It is an amazing feeling

You are radiating brilliance

You are radiating courage

You want to admire the scenery a bit more

You can't get enough of it in your eyes

But it's getting dark

It's time for you to go home

The kids have also started returning to their homes with their sheep

You must also return

But you will be returning victorious

You have conquered your fears

Beyond that fog is your home

Come back

Become aware of your surrounding

Become aware of your breathing

You are doing great

You are feeling completely relaxed

There is no fear now

There is no anxiety

There is no stress

You can open your eyes now

Or choose to sit in this position for a bit longer

Relish the feeling for as long as you want.

Relaxing Self Massage

The objective of this meditation session is to physically release the tension from the body through self-massage and mentally release the tension through meditation. It is going to be a completely relaxing session. You can sit in any comfortable position you want. If you wish you can sit on a chair or even in the cross-legged posture.

Simply follow the guided meditation session and you will feel completely relaxed at the end of it.

Take your position at the place of your meditation

Be seated

Sit in a completely relaxed manner

Don't do anything immediately

Ground yourself first

Just sit completely relaxed for a few minutes

If something important comes to your mind write it down

If there is something that is bothering you, write it down

Get into a comfortable position

Keep your back straight

Ensure that your shoulders are also straight

Your back and neck should be in a straight line

Now, close your eyes

Lean slightly forward and then backward

Lean-to your left side and then to your right

Now, bring yourself to the center and find the best and most comfortable position

Feel your head positioned on your neck

Raise your chin slightly upwards

This will help you in placing your focus between your eyebrows

Try to feel your whole body

Notice if there is tension anywhere

If you feel any part tense, release the tension

Adjust your body to release the pressure

Start by inhaling through your nose

Breathe in deeply

Let the air travel through your body

Feel the areas of tension

Hold the air for a while

Then, release it through your mouth

Your inhalations should be shorter

Your exhalations should be longer

Breathe in

Breathe out

Breathe in the positive energy

Feel the love and compassion

Let your worries dissipate

Don't bother about things much

Simply enjoy the moment

Breathe in

Breathe out

Breathe in

Breathe out

Breathe in

Breathe out

Breathe in

Breathe out

Think of the areas in which you are feeling the stress

Direct your breathing to those areas

Try to release the tension mentally

Breathe in

Breathe out

Breathe in

Breathe out

Now rub your palms together vigorously

This should comfortably heat up your palms

Devote some time to it

Don't rush the process

The longer you rub your palms together

The more energy they will accumulate

They will also get smoother and provide more warmth and good sensation

Now take your index finger and the middle finger of both hands

Use them to touch at the sides of your neck

Start massaging the sides of the neck in a circular motion

Start massaging gently

Move both your fingers in a circular motion

Massage this area for a minute or so

Adjust the pressure you want to apply to the area

You shouldn't press very hard

Gently hold both sides of your neck and massage

Stop after a minute or when you start feeling relaxed

Give yourself some time

Now start pressing under your chin with your thumb

Move your thumb in a circular fashion gently

This action will provide a soothing sensation

Messaging this area will provide a soothing sensation to your whole head

Now, take your index finger and middle finger together again

Press them right below your ear lobes

Move them gently in a circular motion

This will provide a soothing sensation to the back of your neck

Your face would also start getting relaxed

Bring your fingers at the joint of your jaws

Start massaging your jaws in circles

This will help in relaxing your facial muscles

You will feel a great rush of energy here

Repeat the motion for a minute

Relax for a moment

Bring your fingers to the back of your ears

Massage in this area for a bit

This is very relaxing for the back of your head

You will feel utterly relaxed all of a sudden

All the pain and tension goes away

Relax for a moment

Now hold your ears from the top

Gently rub the top of your ears

This is also very soothing and relaxing

You can repeat this motion a few times

Relax for a moment

Now cup your ears completely

Rub your ears in a soft circular motion with your palms

This also feels very soothing

Keep rubbing the ears as long as you feel comfortable

Relax for a moment

Now bring your fingers to your temple

If you are feeling headache, running your temples in a circular motion will help a lot

Simply rub with the tip of your fingers in a gentle circular motion

It releases all the tension that might have built up while messaging the jaws

It will relax your head completely

Relax for a moment

Now put your thumbs at the side of your base bridge

Your thumb should be placed beside the nose bridge and the side of your eyes

Place your index fingers at the top of your forehead together

Now your fingers will be forming a bridge of their own

Start massaging both the points together

This is a very relaxing exercise

You will feel your eyes getting completely relaxed

If you wear glasses, this will be really soothing for you

The glasses put a lot of pressure on the nose bridge that we don't usually realize

Doing this exercise releases that pressure

Now, you can put the index finger and middle finger of one of your hands at the center of your forehead

Place your other hand at the top of your hand

Now move your fingers in a circular motion at your third eye chakra which is at the center of your forehead

This is a very relaxing exercise

The hand placed on the top of your head is supporting your crown chakra

Take deep breaths as you rub the point of your third eye chakra

Be gentle

Press this area for a minute or so

This will relax your mind completely as this point is the seat of your third eye

Your power to sense things improves with this exercise

In the end, you can also massage the back of your head with both your hand

Place your thumbs at the back of your ears

Take your fingers at the back of your head

Now gently rub the back of your head

It will release any kind of tension retained by your head

You will now feel your head completely relaxed

If there is any stress on your shoulders and upper trapezius you can rub these areas too

Cup the shoulders of the opposite sides by your hands

Now move them in a circular motion

This releases the tension in the shoulders

If there is any tension in the upper trapezius

Hold it by your hands and massage it very gently

This will relax your shoulders completely

Now, again focus on your breathing

Breathe in

Breathe out

Breathe in

Breathe out

Breathe in

Breathe out

Relax your body completely and become aware of your surroundings

You will feel completely relaxed and calm.

Chapter 4   Sleep Hypnosis Scripts

Welcome.

This is going to be a thirty-minute guided hypnosis session to help you drift off into a deep and relaxing sleep. The most important thing to do while listening to this session is to keep an open mind. You must go with the flow, listen to my voice, and remember to breathe.

Remember, it is not always possible to enter a light hypnotic state on the first try, but we are going to try as I guide you gently and smoothly into this state so you can fall asleep. Please bear in mind that you are not going to enter any sort of deep catatonic state. Nothing is going to be physically altered within the realm of your mind. The process of hypnosis and this guided meditation is extremely safe, and you are in control of it.

Now, I want you to get comfortable. Because you are trying to achieve a deep sleep, you should be lying down, your head resting on your most comfortable pillow and you are warmed by your softest blanket. Lie back and let your shoulders go slack, relaxing against the cushion of your bed. Gently close your eyes and release all the tension from your muscles. Release the tension in your arms, then your legs. Let go of the tension in your chest and in your back. All of the muscles in your body begin to feel looser and looser and your body is feeling light.

Focus your attention on your toes. Softly wiggle all ten toes once, and then again. Feel the energy released from your movement and the stillness that follows. Your toes are now ready for sleep.

Next, tighten the muscles in your calves and hold for one, two, three seconds. Now release the muscles. Tighten them again for one, two, three seconds. Now release. The excess energy that keeps you up at night has been expelled from your calves. Your calves are now ready for sleep.

Next, squeeze your thigh muscles and hold for one, two, three seconds. Now release. The tension that was once stored there has been released. Your thighs are now ready for sleep. Feel the lightness that has cloaked your legs. Your legs feel weightless as if they could float up to the ceiling.

Focus your attention on your buttocks. Tighten your muscles in buttocks for one, two, three seconds. Now release the muscles. The tightness in your buttocks and lower back has been relieved. Your buttocks and lower back are now ready for sleep.

Focus your attention on your abdomen. Squeeze your abdominal muscles for one, two, three seconds. Now release. The anxiety that has been stored up and deterring sleep has been released. Your abdomen is now ready for sleep.

Concentrate on your chest. Tighten the muscles in your chest for one, two, three seconds. Now release. The sadness that has been weighing on you and preventing your mind from resting has been expelled. Your chest is now ready for sleep.

Direct your attention now to your shoulders. Tighten the muscles in your shoulder for one, two, three seconds. Now release. The stress that has been building in the deep tissue of your shoulders has now been dissolved. Your shoulders are now ready for sleep.

Focus your attention on your neck. Gently tighten the muscles and hold for one, two, three seconds. Now release. Gently tighten the muscles in your jaw and hold for one, two, three seconds. Now release. Gently tighten the muscles in your mouth and hold for one, two, three seconds. Now release. Gently squeeze your eyelids tighter for one, two, three seconds. Now release. The tension that was held in your face has now been released.

The entirety of your body has been washed with serenity as you expel the negative energy from your muscles. Now that your body is relaxed, your mind can now relax in preparation for deep slumber. Realize how free it feels to let go of all built up tension. In this moment nothing else matters. You are free. You are relaxed. You are weightless.

There is nowhere for you to be and you have everything you need. You are here, in this moment, permitting the calming sensation to course through your body. Your thoughts drift away. You don't try to follow or catch them. With each breath you take, you are feeling more and more serene. Breathe in, welcoming peace and harmony to your soul. Breathe out, exhaling all the negative energy and releasing your control. Realize how good it feels to be so relaxed.

Focus on being as relaxed as you can be at this moment. Allow your mind to settle down a little, to quiet, to be still. Instead, focus more on your body. How does it feel lying in your bed? Examine the coziness you feel beneath your sheets. Feel how smooth your sheets are and gentle weight of your blanket on top of you. Relax in the embrace of the softest bed in the world. You are content in every way.

Imagine that on the other side of the room is an open fire crackling. The orange and yellow flames emanate a sensation of calmness as its soft light can be seen upon your walls and ceiling. You feel the warmth of this sensation. You watch closely as the flames flicker and dance upon the logs. The sound of the crackling fire reminds you that you are safe in this space. In this bed you are warm, cozy, and protected.

Scan your body for tension. Find where you still hold stress in your body. Examine your shoulders, your neck, your temples, and your back. Find the stress that is hiding and release it. Allow your body to feel relieved, relaxed, at peace.

Examine the aroma of the fire as it fills the room. The fragrance is deep and musky. It reminds you of good memories with the ones who love you. These memories remind you that your life is beautiful. Place both hands on your stomach, one below your ribs and one above your belly button. Take a deep breath in through your nose, inhale those good memories. Let the air fill your belly and your hands rise on top of your abdomen. Then, through your nose, exhale all of the negativity you have collected. The worries that you harbor are no longer welcome here.

Breathe in the relaxing scent of the fireplace, fill up your stomach like it is a balloon. Let your hands move as your inhale. Then exhale any remaining tension. You now feel loose and at ease. There is a calmness that envelopes your body as you breathe. As you feel more relaxed, you hear only the fire in this quiet space. The quietness of the room also quiets your mind and you welcome rest and relaxation.

As you lay, keep breathing and reveling in this blissful setting: you're tucked inside your cozy bed with a fire to keep you warm. Focus on this serene moment and give yourself permission to enjoy it. Remember that you are in control. Many times, your mind is overthinking, overanalyzing, and too critical. In this moment, it is you who is in control and you will exhale those negative thoughts. As you exhale, you regain your balance and you feel content. Your body feels looser, lighter, and a weight is lifted off your chest.

Your body is light and warm as you listen to my voice. Let me guide you as you drift off. I'm going to count now and you will listen. Let my voice lull you. You are safe and relaxed and warm.

Ten… Your body is entirely loose and relaxed.

Nine… You are in a peaceful, calm, and safe environment.

Eight… You can feel the warmth and love of those who care about you, enveloping your senses.

Seven… The sound of the burning fire, the crackling of wood lulls you further into an even deeper state of relaxation.

Six… You inhale all of the good in the world with each breath you take.

Five… You exhale all the bad, expelling all of your stress and anxiety with each breath out.

Four… You feel your body getting lighter until you are almost like a feather in the breeze.

Three… You feel your mind becoming heavier and brimming with warmth and love.

Two… Accept the peace that has engulfed you, understand that it is good. Let it send you off ever deeper into the feeling of relaxation.

One… You feel yourself drifting all the way down, as deep as you can go, nearer to the bottom, towards warmth and sleep.

You are safe and you are relaxed. Allow yourself to feel safe and relaxed in this space.

Imagine that you are a leaf on a tree. You are connected to a giant colony of other leaves attached to a branch. That branch is attached to a trunk. You are a part of a busy, ever rustling tree. However, you want to be still. You need to rest. You need to separate yourself from the busyness of your world. You decide that you will depart your branch and you begin to float. Slowly, as if gravity has slowed your fall, you twirl and roll in the breeze. You are peacefully drifting further and further, reassured that you are safe.

Instead of the ground, you see that there is a quiet pond below your tree and soon you will touch the surface. As you float towards it, you notice its stillness. There are no ripples or disturbances. The surface is smooth and clear; it is as reflective as a mirror. As you reach the water, you greet the surface with a delicate kiss.

You send gentle, peaceful ripples from your contact. Concentric circles echo out to the edges of the pond. This energy radiates from you until the last ripple falls away. It is now you on the water, undisturbed and immersed in the tranquility of your setting. You drift on the surface of your unconsciousness. You feel the warmth of the water beneath you and surrounding you. The water is so soothing that you feel yourself getting heavier. You feel as though you could keep floating deeper and deeper beneath the surface until you fell asleep.

The relaxation that you feel now is beckoning you closer to rest, to deep sleep. Notice how relaxed you are in this very moment. Notice how soothing the sensations are in your body. Breathe in the relaxation that the water provides. Breathe out any tension you have.

I am going to count down from five. When I reach one, you are going to fully embrace the peace that has engulfed you and lose yourself in sleep. You will feel yourself slipping into a calm and serene rest.

Five… You think of the still surface of the pond, and how it provided safety for you, the leaf. The calm water is summoning your sleep.

Four… You feel the warmth of tranquility ripple from the top of your scalp and down your neck. It glides through your shoulders, radiates through your chest and stomach, and finally glazes over your legs. You are encompassed by this sensation.

Three… You feel your body become heavy and you softly sink in a little deeper to your consciousness. You are safe and protected.

Two… You feel yourself drift away, like your leaf on the still pond. You float away, quietly into the night.

One… You are now asleep, resting and at peace.

Breathe in, breathe out. Breathe in, breathe out. When you wake up, you will be renewed and refreshed and ready to take on the day. You will be ready to conquer the obstacles of your life now that you have conquered sleep.

Chapter 5   Guided Meditation: 30 Minute Deep Sleep Hypnosis for Better Sleep, Stress Relief, & Relaxation

[To be read quite slowly. Increasingly slowly to help bring the more rapid state of waking in line with the rhythmic and slower cadence of breath and sleep]

Welcome.

This meditation is to be experienced lying down in a safe, comfortable and uninterrupted place you can remain asleep once the meditation plays through.

(PAUSE)

Lying down now, give yourself the space to breathe deeply and fully. Allow the breath to enter through your nose, descend along the length of your body and reach your belly which rises in response to the fullness of oxygenated air. It feels SO GOOD to let in this fresh new breath.

As you exhale, let the parts of the day you no longer need rise up and out of your body with your breath, gently breathing out through your mouth, lips shaped into a small "O". Feel the weight of the day leaving your body as you exhale, your belly flattening as the air leaves and pause here in this open space of release.

Good.

Now, breathe again in through your nose, imagining the breath has a color to it, any color of your choosing, the first color that comes to mind. Allow this color to permeate your entire body as you breathe it in through you nose, as the air travels to every single cell, bringing light and warmth, oxygen and peace to your being. You are a being filled with this colored light and infused with the newness of the atmosphere around you, a system of molecules and vibrations always regenerating with its own wisdom. All you must do to be a part of it is to breathe it in. Let it fill you.

Wonderful.

As you exhale, allow everything that no longer serves you to simply rise up and float out of your body through your rounded lips in a nice long exhale. Find yourself noticing the lightness that comes with each breath and release. Feel the peace of letting go the day. The week. The elements in your life you no longer need. How easy it is to simply let them go. How good it feels to breathe in the atmosphere. To take part in the universe. To discover the grace of breath.

Continue now, breathing in through your nose, bringing in light and color and newness and exhaling through the mouth, releasing all that is ready to release.

[1 minute of silence or light music]

Beautiful.

You find yourself feeling lighter by the moment, releasing everything that no longer serves and embracing the expansive wisdom that continually surrounds you, allowing the regenerative nature of the universe to become part of you through breath and rhythm. Through the simple act of breathing. This communion with life all around you. And it feels so good to be part of this rhythm.

Notice also how your body becomes more grounded, more connected to the substrate beneath it, to the earth itself. How you are at once light as air and part of the earth. How you are right where you need to be, in the most perfect place for you right now in this entire universe, supported and free.

And allow yourself to deepen further into this peace. Let any tension remaining in your body, your mind, flow down into the ground, into the core of the earth itself to be transformed and used for other purposes. You do not have to hold onto it any longer. The earth itself knows how to best use the excess energies we do not need.

Feel yourself melt right into the place you are, becoming fluid, becoming more sentient, becoming grace. Movement and light, breath and air. Every part of you now, every cell in your body breathes in the universe around you and breathes out in communion. Breathing becomes– you realize it IS– a conversation. It is a connection. Breathing is BEING life.

You are being. You are life. You are in the perfect place at the perfect time. You are everything you need to be right now.

Your body is pleasurably connected to the fibers beneath you. You notice the pleasant heaviness that comes from the safety of sinking into a warm space, a space you can trust, a space in which you are completed connected, held and supported. With every breath now, you sink deeper and deeper into a state of peace, of ultimate comfort, of knowing your place in the world. It is as simple as this, a noticing of the way you are part of everything around you and the beauty that comes from breathing in the atmosphere and breathing out the colors of your breath to create a resonance that holds and supports you right where you are at; just as you are now.

Every time you exhale now you create a field of light and color around you. Every time you inhale, the light and color becomes part of you. Every time you inhale, you feel yourself fill with lightness of air. Every time you exhale, you deepen into the fibers below you and the support of the earth itself.

Allow your noticing to grow larger.

Notice how the room around you becomes filled with this positive light and energy that you are breathing in and out. How the energies of the entire universe, how the support and grounding of the earth infuses the space in which you find yourself, and how this changes the space itself. Fills it with more peace, more safety, more comfort, more life and love.

Allow this to expand even further. Notice how this beautiful energy also infuses the entire house or building, the larger area in which you find yourself. How your very nexus, your very center of breathing and imbibing the universe is helping the entire space around you, large and small, near and far, become more infused with loving, peaceful and serene energy. How you create a larger sphere of radiance that surrounds as far as you can see, as far as you can feel, and breathes with you, within you.

[1 minute music/silence]

Ahhhh (sigh type of voice, in order to engage this response in listener, like a long deep exhale). This is the majesty of the living world as it becomes part of you, responds to you, emanates from you. This is the magic of breath and grounding. This is your deepest nature, your connected being, your beautiful soul. At once a part of everything around you and helping to create that which is around you.

Each breath continues to deepen your state of peace and harmony, rest and relaxation, trust and security in the communication you have with the particles of air, the elements of nature, the energies of the universe.

As with a cradle, you are held and supported, loved and carried and can allow yourself to sink deeper into a state of bliss and union, comfort and support.

You notice the colors shift and change, the sounds soften and swell, the concrete pieces of waking life fall away. The world blends and melds with your larger sense of being, with the larger consciousness of the earth, with the wisdom of the universe at large. Your body softens and stretches, settles and soothes. You are fluid and warm, bathed by the universe itself as you drift into a restful state of existence.

Let the rhythm of your breath soothe you. Feel its rise and fall in its most natural state massaging every cell in your body. Massaging the musculature surrounding your skull, releasing the tensions on the bones, your jaw, your eyes, your sinuses and tongue entirely. Feel the sweet release of open space for your mind to flow freely, your head itself swoon. Let your head sway side to side as you continue to unwind down into the neck, releasing even further any aches or pains, any stiffness and tightness, becoming fluid, light, air, becoming oxygen itself flowing through the body, connecting to the space around you.

Let your shoulders drop into the surface beneath you, releasing every bit of weight they carry and your chest rise and fall easily in the softness you create with your breath. It is as though effortless, your breathing, your releasing, your increasing sense of peace and comfort. This restful state of bliss.

Notice your abdomen soften, with each and every breath, your belly is massaged from the inside out, your entire body can sense the renewed vigor of the cells, so full of oxygen and the softness this release brings. Even your hips roll wide open, released into the rhythm of the breath, the flow of blood and openness of your state of being.

Your low back and legs follow suit, settling into the most comfortable state of repose, rocking slightly with each intake of breath and settling with each outtake until your exhale reaches the very tips of your toes, the base of your feet and sends itself out into the air around you, out into the universe to be recycled, regenerated, and transformed into new energy or matter. You exhale all that you no longer need and inhale the freshness of new breath, the lightness of being, the fluidity of an ever nourishing universe.

When you inhale again, you revel in the lightness of your body, the sense of being water itself, the motion of being still. You find you are everything that is peaceful about this universe, that you are so satisfied in this state of being. That you have become peace itself.

Your body knows how to best support you. It knows how to hold the attention of deep relaxation while being alert to the world around you. Your mind knows how to heed the call of the body, the need for rest, the ability to transition between states. It knows that when it is needed it will be called upon again, but for now, everything is just fine. There is nothing but this space, nothing but this peace, and a certainty in the wisdom of dreams.

You float and absorb the energies of the womb of life and allow yourself the regenerative nature of sleep knowing that anything important will gain your attention as it needs to, you need not hold onto any ideas or thoughts, they will find you again when it is time.

And in this you drift and know this is a type of home. A connection to the cosmos inside of you and all around you. A colorful and flavorful connection to life that blends with your cells, blends with you neurons and leads you into a blissful form of serenity conducive to sleep.

Breathe now, in and out at your own pace, while the energies of the universe move through you, cleanse you, inform you, hold and support you and allow you the deep healing of rest. Feel the incredible expansiveness and drift of the universe in your cells and in your peaceful body. Allow yourself to sink in.

[Music/sounds to support the transitional state into sleep. Next 15-20minutes]

[Towards ends of the recording, leave with this whispered prompt]

As the music fades you find yourself sinking even deeper into rest. The silence brings you a peace greater than you have known and carries you in sleep for exactly the right amount of time for you.

You breathe and find peace in being.

You are exactly where you need to be.

You are just perfect as you are.

You continue to breathe and release.

As the world too, breathes and unfolds.

Chapter 6   Better Sleep Habits

Sleep is not about just what happens at night. You need to live a healthy life throughout your day in order to get the right kind of sleep needed. This meditation is going to be all about guiding you through the healthiest habits needed throughout the day. They will be filled with affirmations that will help you emphasize the importance of implementing these habits in your life.

Meditation for Better Sleep Habits

Getting a good night's sleep can start the moment that you wake up.

This guided meditation is going to take you through an entire day, reiterating the most important sleep habits that you'll need to include in your regimen.

This is a meditation that can be done at any time during the day. You will still want to ensure that you are in a safe place so that if you do happen to drift off, it is okay to do so. However, this is not one that should only be performed at night. You can do it whenever you want a reminder of the healthy habits that you need to include in your life.

This is going to be a visual meditation. You will envision all that needs to be done in a day in order to direct your attention towards making sure that you will get a good night's sleep at the end of the day.

In order to clear your mind and get you relaxed, start with a basic breathing exercise. Start by breathing in through your nose for five, and out through your mouth for five. We are going to do this three times in a row.

Start by breathing in for one, two, three, four, five. And out for six, seven, eight, nine, ten.

Do this again for one, two, three, four, and five. Feel as your breath comes out for six, seven, eight, nine, and ten.

Then breathe in for one, two, three, four, and five. Finally, breathe out for a third time for six, seven, eight, nine, and ten.

Now your breathing has become regulated and it will be much easier to focus on the guided meditation.

Start by thinking about what you do every morning. This will usually involve the initial wake-up period.

You have to focus on waking up early enough to give you time to relax before you have to start the day.

Rushed wakeups will keep us feeling rushed throughout the rest of our day. As you breathe in, think of all the times that you have been late to something. As you breathe out, remind yourself that you will not let this happen anymore. You need to start to focus on healthy sleeping habits in order to ensure that you are getting a proper amount of rest every night. This will include waking up on time.

Think now about a life where you eat healthy and get a little exercise as well. The food that you eat will determine how you will feel at night.

The amount you move your body throughout the day will play into how you are able to fall asleep at night.

Start to focus on the better habits that you can implement into your life in order to align with what needs to be done to get a good night's sleep.

Remember that the choices you make regarding what food you decide to eat is going to directly affect how it feels when you fall asleep.

The things that go into your body become a part of you. Create a body that will be energized throughout the day so that you can wake up peacefully.

As you breathe in, take in all of the old habits that you have that might have been hindering your good night's sleep. As you breathe out, let go of all the unhealthy decisions that you might have made in the past. As you breathe out, realize that you do not have to partake in these bad habits anymore.

Picture yourself in a place where you are always tired. Maybe this is your office, a classroom, or somewhere else.

How do you feel when you are there? Imagine that this place is surrounding you now.

As you breathe in, take in your surroundings. As you breathe out, breathe that life into all that surrounds you. What does this place look like? What about it makes you feel tired?

Now imagine being here and being completely energized. Imagine that you are able to stay awake and alert.

Imagine that you are energized, refreshed, and ready for whatever might be waiting for you.

You have the ability to do this. The chance to be refreshed, awake, and focused is all in your hands.

As you breathe in, take in the realization that you are in charge of your life.

Accept that you have some new healthier habits that you need to focus on adding to your life.

Each time you breathe out, let go of your past. Separate yourself from the decisions that you've made in the past that weren't in the best interest of your healthy sleep pattern.

You can put an emphasis going forward on getting better sleep. When your sleep is balanced, so will everything else in your life.

When you take care of one aspect of your health, the rest will fall into place. In order to live a harmoniously healthy life, you must put a focus on getting the right amount of sleep.

Continue to practice these validating breathing exercises on a daily basis. This is a good reminder to carry with you that you need to emphasize sleep for health, and nothing else.

We are going to transition into some affirmations going forward that will help drive home the idea of better sleep for your health.

Focus on the way your body is feeling now that it is more relaxed.

Breathe in for one, two, three, four, five, and out for six, seven, eight, nine, and ten.

Breathe in again for one, two, three, four, five, and finally out again for six, seven, eight, nine, and ten.

You are now much more relaxed than you were before. You are focused on implementing healthier habits and making the right choices for your sleeping life. You can either do another sleep meditation to drift off into sleep or move onto affirmations to help remember what is most important about your health – getting the right sleep.

Chapter 7   Deep Sleep Hypnosis - Sleepy Ocean Visualization

It is going to be a really nice sleep tonight…before you fall asleep, I will take you to the most beautiful beach you've ever seen. This place will relax you and calm you to your very soul.

First, take a nice deep breath, getting into a very comfortable position. Rest your head upon your soft pillow and take another deep breath…relaxing into the bed, loosening all muscles.

Breathing deeply, letting your legs relax and sink into the bed…breathe fully, letting your torso melt into the mattress…breathing, completely let go the muscles in your neck and shoulders, letting you head be cradled by the pillow…take one last deep and relaxing breath, as you exhale let your eyes gently close.

Good…

Relax your body even more by letting go of any areas of tension…breathe in again slowly… release the air with a whooshing sound, like a wave crashing on the sand…

Become more and more relaxed with each breath…

Breathe in again very slowly…pause for a moment….and let it go…

Feel your body giving up all tension…becoming fully relaxed…enjoying every moment of this calm and peaceful breathing…

There is a gentle wave of relaxation flowing through your body…down and up…up and down…just like the waves of the great ocean…

It flows from the tips of your toes, through your feet, up your ankles, and lower legs… through the knees, thighs, hips and pelvis…the relaxation flows through your abdomen, chest, back and shoulders…down each arm, relaxing any tension…all the way to the hands and each fingertip…it flows up your neck, relaxing you deeply…the back of your head fully relaxes, your facial muscles let go completely…and the very top of your head, including your brain, becomes deeply relaxed…

Breathe in slowly and deeply again…releasing the air with a whooshing sound…and as you do bring into your mind the thought of a white sand beach.

The sand is warm…and as soft as velvet under your feet…

The waves of the turquoise ocean in front of you is making that gentle whooshing sound, just like your breath…

This beach is surrounded by tropical forest. You can hear the song of beautiful birds being carried through the air…you notice the leaves on the palm trees are moving with the wind, making a soothing rustling sound…you can hear crickets and tropical frogs enjoying their life in the rainforest.

Notice the different greens of the nature, the beauty in the way that each leaf reflects the sunlight.

You can feel the gentle warmth of the sun on your skin, relaxing you. This place is the definition of tranquility. The ocean water is shallow for a distance, then far out along the horizon you can see the water gets deeper and is therefore a deep sapphire blue.

There are white fluffy clouds in the sky that resemble the blossom of cotton in its raw form…drifting by, slowly in the sky. The sun's rays alternate between warming your skin and being hidden behind the passing clouds.

The beach sand turns into giant rocks to your left, that soar into tall caves along the water's edge. As you walk towards these caves, you feel the sand moving under each footstep…you gaze behind you and see a long strand of your footprints trailing behind you. The rock formations get more massive as you draw closer… as you draw near the cave, you find yourself under the shadow of its cliff, and the air becomes cool from the shade.

There is a large opening in the rocks… it is a welcoming entrance.

As you go inside the cave, you can hear the sounds of the ocean waves become amplified as they bounce off the rock walls. This cave is magnificent. You can hear the sounds of trickling water, so you follow it to find its source. Along the interior wall of the cave, fresh water is springing from rocks, making the most relaxing sound of moving water you've ever heard. This water seems to glow, although there is no sunlight reflecting in the cave, it shimmers with light before your eyes.

You cup your hands together and gather some of this water, bringing it to your lips for a drink. It is the purest and refreshing water you have ever tasted. It nourishes and replenishes you… hydrating every part of your being with its beauty.

The tropical birds know of this water source, and make their way flying into the cave, chirping their beautiful song. There are all different types of birds, large and small. They land on the floor of the cave and drink the fresh water that is collected in various puddles below. Bringing their beaks down, scooping the water, then raising their heads high to allow the water to trickle down their throats. They are not afraid of you; it is almost as if you are part of their flock.

These magnificent birds are co close, you can clearly see the beautiful rainbow of colors that make up their feathers… bright reds… yellows… greens… and turquoise blues that match the water of the ocean…. Their eyes are surrounded by the crisp white of their skin, and they look directing at you with kindness and curiosity… After getting their fill of hydrating water, they fly out of the cave and back into the rainforest.

You take a moment to sit down in this cave, there is the perfect shape rock protruding from the ground that almost resembles a bench. Have a seat and close your eyes for a moment, tuning into the sounds around you….

The waves… the distant birds… the tricking fresh water… the breeze… each sound soothes you to your very soul… take a deep breath in and hear the sound of the air going in and out of your lungs… you can smell the clean salt water…

(pause)

Open your eyes and see the cave towering above you… What a beautiful spot.

You are ready to go back out and explore the beach, because it has gotten a little cool for you here…

As you make your way out of the cave, the cool rock under your feet turns back into sand… you pass into the sunlight and feel the sunrays begin to nourish your skin. The water is so clear and inviting that you decide to go for a little swim. The sand becomes firmer under your feet because it is saturated with sea water… a waves comes closer and catches your feet. At first, the water seems cool, but it's actually the perfect temperature. The waves rush up to your ankles, and your feet are being buried in the sand as your weight presses you down into the earth.

You make your way into the water and can see that it is shallow for a long distance. It goes to just above your waist. Curious to see what's going on below the surface, you decide to dip your head under the water…. As you do, you find that allowing yourself to become weightless in the ocean is one of the most serene experiences in your life.

Without hesitation, you open your eyes underwater to find that you can see perfectly clear, without any discomfort.

In front of you, there is an immaculate reef, teeming with fish. You swim closer, finding that you don't have an urgency to go up for air. It is almost as if you are a tropical fish in this ocean.

As you swim closer to this city of underwater life, you see that the colors are more brilliant that anything on land. It's as almost as if you are witnessing the rainbow manifesting as life. Everything you see is alive… moving in the ocean's gentle current…

A few small yellow fish with black stripes notice your arrival… they look at you with curiosity in their eyes, and excitement in their swimming. Then they travel back down into a giant pink sea anemone… you can see that this is their home. Several yellow fishes pop in and out of the living home, dancing about… it's almost as if they are showing off their place of residence.

A large purple fish with bright glowing green spots catches your eye… swimming slowly by with confidence and grace… They notice you, but don't seem to be phased by your appearance…

You are witnessing every color you can possibly imagine in your view of this reef… from the blackness of the pupils of the swimming creatures, to the shimmering white light of the sun cascading through the water like a diamond prism.

Everything is peaceful here at the shallow reef.

You are about ready to head back to the shore to enjoy a walk through the sand… then you suddenly see a mighty sea turtle coming close by… the way their arms and legs push them through the water makes the turtle weightless, though you know he could easily weigh more than you. The sweetness in their eyes comforts you to the soul…

Just when you thought this experience couldn't get any better, you see there is a trail of baby turtles following behind… you thought by the size of this sea turtle, it was a male, but now you can see the gentleness that could only be embodied by a caring mother. Her hatchlings have made the daunting journey into the expansive ocean. They are vibrant and ready to take on life. This is only the beginning of a long lifetime along the reef.

You are grateful for this experience in the reef, and it's time to head back to the beach. Getting out of the water is effortless because the waves are gentle, and the water is shallow.

The sun begins drying your skin…. the clouds are passing by ever so slowly… you are beginning to feel tired from taking in all the beauty around you, and just so happens that a plush beach recliner is positioned facing the water, with a large white umbrella providing just the right amount of shade…

Have a seat and position yourself on the chair so that all of your muscles can let go… you are fully ready to take a long nap in this paradise. Inhale deeply the sweetness of the air… exhale into complete tranquility… hear the nature behind you…. The ocean in front of you… and the breeze all around you….

You see the cave you were exploring earlier in the distance and can remember the crisp taste of the fresh spring water…

You can feel the cushioned beach chair supporting you… Every part of your body and mind are at peace, and deeply relaxed…

Gazing out upon the big blue, you notice the horizon, and how it is the only perfectly straight line in the landscape… You enjoy the precision of how the ocean meets the sky.

Take in a few more deep breaths as you lazily keep your eyes open enjoying the sights of this beach paradise.

Breathing in deeply… relaxing more and more… exhale into serenity…

Breathing in fully… let your body sink down, melting any last bit of tension away… exhale into tranquility…

Continue breathing slowly… Allowing the breath to lull you into a deep sleep… slowing down more and more….

You can hear the sounds of the waves gently crashing on the sand… in and out… as the waves come and go, just like your breath…

Allow your eyes to gently close as you rest on your beach chair…

You sleep deeply and soundly… fully rejuvenating as the hours pass by… sleeping this well comes easily to you… you let everything go, so that you get the restful sleep you deserve…

Letting each breath relax you even more… taking you into a deep, deep sleep.

Good.

Allow your mind to drift and wander to wherever it takes you… into the dream world… where there are endless possibilities for you to learn and grow…

Allow my voice to fade into the distance now as you drift off to sleep…

Goodnight…

Chapter 8   Deep Sleep Techniques

Whether you find it difficult to sleep at night as a result of stress, tiredness, work or several other factors, or you find your sleep unsatisfactory, you might be suffering from insomnia. Insomnia is commonly called difficulty falling asleep, or staying awake, and there two types of insomnia.

Acute insomnia is mostly caused as a result of lifestyle, or circumstances. A security officer on night duty will find it difficult to fall asleep on duty, likewise a first-time dad may find it difficult to fall asleep thinking of his precious wife in labor.

While, chronic insomnia is a complicated type of insomnia. There is no known underlying cause, yet the individual finds it difficult to either fall asleep, or sleep at night for long hours. Such person may also experience disrupted sleep, for more than 3 times a week.

Experiencing insomnia regularly causes mood disturbances, fatigue, stress and difficulty concentrating. Although, insomnia can be caused by factors like anxiety, work related stress, lifestyle, and sicknesses. However, the approach to overcome insomnia is not easy for some persons, yet there is one possible way to overcome not just insomnia but enjoy a long, satisfactory sleep for the rest of your life.

How Does Meditation Cure Insomnia

Meditation is a relaxation technique worth trying, which can help improve your sleep, make you fall asleep easily and also make your sleep satisfactory, such that you wake up feeling refreshed. Meditation harmonizes the mind and body, and also influences the brain and the way it functions. The effect of meditation on your mind and body is that you become calm, and relaxed afterwards.

Effect of Meditation on Insomnia

During meditation, the mind is focused on one thing, which prevents the mind from wandering. Your mind and thoughts are brought to the now moment during meditation. Hence, anxiety disappears and it becomes easier to fall asleep.

During the meditation, your mind and body are been connected to each other, and they both become relaxed and calm, which helps you sleep as soon as you get in bed.

Furthermore, meditation helps boost the hormone called melatonin that regulates the sleep and wake cycle. Without stress, the melatonin level is usually at its peak at night to ensure you get a sound, and restful sleep. However, the presence of stress among other factors that causes insomnia, the melatonin level drastically reduces, thereby insomnia occurs. With meditation, the melatonin level increases because stress has been reduced, and the body is in a relaxed state.

Meditation Techniques for Insomnia

If you want to experience an undisrupted sleep, an intense meditation must be done frequently. There are different techniques of meditating for insomnia and understanding process help us to get started immediately.

- Cognitive shuffling

Cognitive shuffling is a simple meditation technique that can be done alone. It is simply a do-it-yourself technique that shuffles your thoughts to sleep. Here is how cognitive shuffling works, when you lie on your bed, your mind is likely to be filled with different thoughts from your daily activities. You can be worried, and anxious about your bills, relationship, the next day activities, such that you find it difficult to fall asleep. The effect of this shuffling on the brain is it tricks the mind to get into a dreaming state.

Tips to Practice Cognitive Shuffling

- Firstly, getting in bed is important

- Right there on your bed, avoid focusing your concerns. Let your deadline be, the bills, the complicated issue at work. Let it all be.

- Now that your mind is free from your fears and worries, create a new engagement like imagining objects, places, names or movies to meditate on. You can imagine different things, like a teddy bear, a fish, a dog, the sky, the rainbow, or the ocean. Note that, the items you are imagining should not be threatening or scary. For instance, instead of imagining an ocean because you have the fear of water, you can imagine the rainbow or the sky with beautiful stars.

- Ensure your eyes are closed before you begin the cognitive shuffling process.

- Process should be repeated if you are still awake, until you run out of words.

- Sa Ta Na Ma (Mantra)

Sa Ta Na Ma is a powerful meditation technique that works on the brain and its functions to reduce risk of depression and other mental illness. It is a mantra that is usually recited in 3 voices; the singing voice which stands for the action voice.

The whispered voice which stands for your inner voice, and

The silent voice is known as your spirit's voice.

SA TA NA MA chant describes the evolutionary aspect of the universe. Each word in the chant has a meaning.

SA means the beginning.

TA means existence and creativeness

NA means death or the end of life

MA means rebirth

The effect of this mantra is displayed by a balance in emotions, and a settled mind.

Practical steps to Sa Ta Na Ma

- Find a comfortable position. You can sit down or lie down.

- Decide on how many minutes you want to recite the mantra.

- Breathe in and out through your nose and mouth and ensure you sigh after this breathing exercise is heard.

- Close your eyes properly, and place your hands either on your lap, or knee. Make sure your palm is facing up.

- Begin chanting slowly, and press the thumb of your hands, with your four fingers. Count your fingers each starting from the thumb to recite the mantra.

- Keep reciting the chant as a calm and slow pace

During recitation, you have to follow the principles of the mantra.

When you mention SA, you count from your index to your thumb

You count from your middle finger to your thumb when you sing TA

You count from your ring finder to thumb when you recite NA

And final you should count from your pinky finger to the thumb when you mention MA.

- Still in that position, sing SA TA NA MA in a loud voice, your voice should be audible, and ensure you move each of your fingers with each sound. The more you sing, the more you feel relaxed and energetic. However, your soul and spirit should feel relaxed and enjoy the sensation which is moving through your body and mind.

- When you feel relaxed, shift your focus and start singing in a whisper voice. At this point, energy is flowing through the body, waist, and knee.

- Next, be focused on silence. Continue counting your fingers and silently repeat the mantra to yourself.

- After singing the mantra completely, breathe in and breathe out with your arms wide open, and lift the hand above your head. Release your hands down, and exhale again. Repeat process until you feel refreshed or drowsy.

What to Expect When Meditating To Fall Asleep

Your expectations when meditating to fall asleep is most likely to have a sound and deep sleep at night, except you are uncertain about the benefits of meditation. Meditation for sleep is similar to other kind of meditation; however, the approach to each of these meditations is what matters.

When meditating, your meditation technique determines what you will have to do. Albeit, you can start preparing for your meditation exercise, by breathing in and out, lying flat on your back. If you are having a guided meditation, all you need to do is follow the instructions instead of been worried about what to do and what not to do.

Furthermore, all you should when meditating to fall asleep is sleep, but try to avoid any form of distractions.

How to Meditate Before Sleep

There are two ways you can meditate before going to bed, it can be a mindful meditation where you pay more attention to your body and mind, and also having a guided meditation where someone leads you through the process of meditation.

Mindfulness meditation can be done alone, in your own room house and house. While guided meditation is a very easy meditation, it is just for you to follow and listen to instructions from a guide.

Guided Meditation Tips for insomnia

Guided meditation is the form of meditation you engage in with the help of a tutor, or instructor. Ensure that you will not be disturbed, during the course of this meditation.

- Lay down on your back, preferably on your bed or mat. Make sure you are comfortable on whatever you are lying on.

- Close your eyes and prepare your mind for the meditation you are about to engage in.

- Breathe in and out, ensure that your breathing out is audible such that it looks like you breathing out heavily. Make your body feel the heaviness, after which your body will be relaxed.

- Pay more attention to your breathing, and you feel easiness. A natural breathing processes.

- At this point, you will feel your body is relaxed. Feel the way your breath travels through your lungs, and hold your breath. As this is happening, you will begin to feel relaxation in your body.

- You can begin to breathe normally right now, and as you breathe you feel your muscles, joints, and back relaxed.

- Pay more attention to your stomach area right now, where your abdominal muscles are present. Tighten the muscles in your abdomen, and hold your breath for 10 seconds and release your muscles. During this release, feel the difference the tightness of your abdominal muscle and the relaxation of these muscles.

- Repeat the above process 5 times.

- Breathe in and out, tighten your abdomen and release it to relaxation.

Feet

- Divert your attention to your feet, and make them relaxed. The relaxation should be from your toes to your ankles. Tighten your toes and feet, and feel them become heavy and relaxed.

- Focus on your nails, feel them relaxed and let go.

- Pay attention to your thigh area, and feel them relaxed.

- Again, focus on your waist, lower and upper back, joints and feel them relaxed. You will feel the feel heavy, and very relaxed

Upper limbs

- At this point, focus your attention on your arms. Feel them heavy and relaxed.

- Get a sense of how heavy your arm is, and feel the relaxation shift to your elbow, wrist, and fingers become very relaxed.

Face, neck and facial muscles

- Shift your focus to your facial muscles, neck and face.

- Every muscle in your face, your cheeks and chin becomes relaxed, and your entire body is now relaxed.

A deeper meditation for the abdomen

- Locate your center, which is your abdominal region. Imagine there is a bowl on your abdomen. Slowly see the bowl rolling over your abdomen area, and it relaxes every muscle the bowl rolls in contact with.

- The bowl now moves slowly from your abdomen area to your right hip carefully and softly massaging the muscles of the hips it comes in contact to.

- Massaging back and forth all the muscles in your abdomen.

- The ball continues to roll over to your knee, and around your knee. You can feel the tension on your navel melting away. Roll the ball slowly to your toe, and over to your toes, from your small toes to the big toes.

Every part of your body this ball comes in contact with feel the part of your body relaxing.

- Now feel the ball begins to roll upwards away from your toes again. Massaging and reducing tension around your toes, knees, ankles and rolls over to your center, your abdominal area.

- Again, this balls rolls to your left thigh, and your knee, massaging both the back and front of your knee.

With your ball you move this ball to wherever you choose, and how long you want it to be.

- With this ball, massage your knee, and ankle and toes. This ball touches every muscle in your toes, it gently massages them and at this point, you feel your muscle relax.

- Feel the ball roll back up your leg, your knee and thigh muscle and arriving back at your center.

- Shift the focus of the ball to the base of your spinal cord. Allow the ball rest there for 5 seconds, and allow it move up your spine, and near your heart. At this point, you can feel the ball massaging the internal organs in your body. The ball massages the heart, and you feel relaxed.

- The ball rolls to your throat area, and the back of your neck area. You feel your neck area relaxing after the ball massages it. You feel tension reducing around your neck area.

- The ball travels down your arm, and to your wrist. The ball gently massages your wrist, and fingers.

- You feel the ball roll up your arm, to your shoulder and neck. It travels down to your elbow, forearm, and wrist and into the palm of your hands.

- Allow the ball gently massage your palm, and fingers. The ball moves up your arm, shoulder and face and as it reaches up in your face, the ball splits into a hundred tiny balls. You feel them travel around your face, to your eyes, eyebrow, cheeks, chin, teeth, tongue and teeth.

- You feel the ball massaging your face and every part of your face. At this point, you should enjoy this facial massage.

- I want you to imagine as you are lying down the ceiling of your house. Your eyes is still closed, so imagine the ceiling of your room opening itself up, and the roof also opens itself open.

- Still looking at this opening, you will see the beautiful white sky. The sky is clear, bright, and the moon is out and also full, filled with stars. This is a magical peaceful night. You are alone, safe in the beautiful part of your house.

- Watch the twinkling and beautiful little stars, looking down on you and you are enjoying the peace of the night.

- You look again at the stars again, the little ones that are thousands of miles away are not shining so beautiful like the big star closer to you, that is looking at you directly from the sky.

- You are looking deep into galaxy, beyond time, you see a million other stars waiting for you and shining at you.

- Take a deep breath. breathe in a rich air from the infinite and beautiful galaxy filled with stars.

- Feel yourself been a part of these stars, there is no separation between you and them. Feel you are already a part of this wonderful galaxy.

- As you experience this, you become a shooting star, shining across the galaxy like others.

- Slowly you begin to fade into the sky, into the unending space and galaxy.

- You are living in the wonders of this space, where there is neither time, past or future. You feel you are the stars, the moon, and you occupy the pace between the planets.

- You are floating off slowly, as you travel across this universe; you feel your body wants to drift away. You feel peace, wholeness, and love.

- When you are ready, and feel relaxed, you can let go of the galaxy. When you drift off, you will drift into a peaceful and wonderful sleep.

Chapter 9   Sleep Meditation

This final meditation in this set is one that is going to help you fall asleep instantly. It is a quicker and shorter meditation that will take you through the visualization exercise.

This process makes it easier for your mindset to go from one where you might be thinking of specific things in your life to a place where you can get into a more dreamlike trance. You will be able to easily fall asleep and get that deep rest you need in order to conquer the day tomorrow. Again, ensure that you are in a comfortable place where you will be able to fall asleep for several hours at a time. This is best at night but if you plan on taking a rather long nap you could do this as well. Keep an open mind and focus on your breathing.

Meditation for a Deep and Quick Sleep

Sleep is incredibly important, but sometimes falling asleep can be difficult if we are not in the right mindset.

For this activity, we are going to take you through a visualization that will help ensure that you can get a deep sleep. It's important before falling asleep to relax your mind so that you can travel gently throughout your brain.

Start off by noticing your breath. Breathe in through your nose and out through your mouth. This is going to help calm you down so that you are able to breathe easier.

Begin by breathing in for five and out for five as we count down from twenty. Once we reach one, your mind will be completely clear. Each time a thought passes in, you will think of nothing. You will have nothing in your sight, and you will only think with your mind.

Make sure that you are in a comfortable place where you can sink into the space around you. Let your body become heavy as it falls into the bed. Keep your eyes closed and see nothing in front of you but darkness.

Each time a thought comes in, keep pushing it away. Breathe in through your nose and out through your mouth.

Remember to breathe in for five and out for five. Keep an empty mind and be ready to travel through a journey that will take you to a restful place.

20, 19, 18, 17, 16, 15, 14, 13, 12, 11, 10, 9, 8, 7, 6, 5, 4, 3, 2, 1

You see nothing in front of you, it is completely dark and you feel your body lifting gently up like a feather. You are light against the bed, and nothing is keeping you down. Continue to feel your body rise higher and higher. You are floating in space. There's black nothingness around you. You are gently drifting around.

You can see a few stars dotting the sky so far away, but for the most part, you see nothing. You feel yourself slowly moving through space. Your body is light and free, and nothing is keeping you strapped down. You're not afraid in this moment.

You are simply feeling easy and free. Breathe in and out, in and out.

You start to drift more towards a few planets, throughout your journey in space. You can really see now that you are up in the highest parts of the galaxy. You see out of the corner of your eye that you can actually catch a glimpse of Earth. You start gently floating towards it, having to put no effort in at all as your body is like a space rock floating through the stars.

Nothing is holding you down.

Nothing is violently pushing you either. Everything that you feel is a gentle and free emotion. You get closer and closer to Earth now and can see all the clouds that surround you. You start to move down, and you gently enter into the cloud area. Normally gravity would pull you down so fast, but right now you're just simply a gentle body drifting through the air. You get closer and closer to the land. You can see some birds here and there and a few cars and lights on the ground beneath you.

You pass all of this. Gently floating over a sleepy town.

Look down and let your mind explore what is it that you see down there. What is it that is in front of your eyes? What do you notice about this world around you as you continue to go closer and closer to home?

You are gently drifting throughout the sky. You can see trees beneath you. Now, if you reached your hand down, you'd even be able to gently feel a few leaves on the tops of the tallest trees. You don't do this now because you're just concerned with continuing to float through the sky. That's all that you really care about in this moment.

You're getting closer and closer and closer to home now, almost ready to fall asleep. You start to see that there is a lake.

You gently float down to the surface of the lake, and you land right in a boat. Your body is a little bit heavier now. You feel it relax into the bottom of the boat. Nothing around you is concerning you right now. You feel no stress or tension in any part of your body. You are simply floating through this space now.

The boat starts to gently drift on the lake. It is dark out now and you look up and see all the stars in the sky. All of this reminds you of the place that you were just a few moments ago. You start to drift closer and closer to sleep.

Do you feel as the tension leaves your body? You are peaceful throughout. You are not holding on to anything that causes you stress or anxiety. You are at ease in this moment. Everything feels good and you have no fear. You drift around in the water now for a little bit longer. You can see everything so clearly in this night sky. Just because it is dark does not mean that it's hard to see. The moon casts a beautiful glow over everything around you. You can feel the moon charging your skin. As you drift closer and closer to sleep, you feel almost nothing in your body now. You continue to focus on your breathing. You are safe, and you are at peace. You are calm, and you are relaxed. You feel incredible in this moment.

The boat starts to lift from the water. You feel as it gets higher above the water. You are even heavier now. Now you are completely glued to this comfortable surface as the boat starts to fly through the sky. You can look down and see that the city beneath you has drifted to sleep. You're getting closer and closer to home now. You can actually see your home beneath you. The boat gently takes you to your front door, and you float right in. No need to walk or climb stairs. You simply float in and straight to your bed.

You fall delicately into your bed with your head resting nicely on a pillow.

Here you are, in this moment, so peaceful and so relaxed. You are completely at ease. There's nothing that stresses you out or causes any anxiety or tension now. You are simply a body that is trying to fall asleep.

As we count down from 20, you will drift off to sleep. You will be in a very relaxed state where nothing stresses you out. You're not concerned with things that happened in the past, and you aren't going to stay up in fear of what might happen tomorrow, you are asleep. You are relaxed.

Breathe in and out. Breathe in and out.

20, 19, 18, 17, 16, 15, 14, 13, 12, 11, 10, 9, 8, 7, 6, 5, 4, 3, 2, 1

Chapter 10   Meditation for Stress Relief

This meditation is a basic one that will help relieve your stress. It is a visualization meditation, where you will be taken through a small journey. You will be able to come out of this with a light feeling and an airy mind that gives you the clarity needed to get the right things done.

Stress Relieving Meditation

It's time to go on a journey. At the beginning of this journey, you are somebody who is filled with stress. The stress keeps you awake at night to the point where you can't even fall asleep anymore. This is not who you're going to be by the end of the journey.

By the end of the journey, you're going to be incredibly tired. You will be so relaxed, that the only thing that you can do is think about closing your eyes and falling asleep. No longer are you going to allow yourself to be awake all night thinking of terrible things that might pass through your head. Rather than focusing on the bad, we are going to be looking at the good. You are going to be stronger and braver at the end of this. The stress relief is going to help you be as relaxed as possible. You will feel good not only when going to bed, but throughout your entire day.

Pick somewhere now where you can be completely calm and relaxed. You can be lying in bed ready to drift away to sleep, or you can simply be sitting in your backyard enjoying the nature around you. Wherever you are, ensure that you can be completely at peace. Remove all distractions, any noise, or anything else that is going to keep you pulled from this meditation and stuck in the moment that's surrounding you. Start to notice the way that you're breathing. Breathe in for a few moments and then breathe out. Breathe in, breathe out.

Feel the air come in through your nose and let it leave through your mouth. This is a common way to practice breathing so that you can be more relaxed. You don't have to do this just when you want to go to bed. You can do this at any moment when you want to bring calmer and serenity into your life. Close your eyes and make sure all thoughts leave your mind. Anytime a thought passes through your mind, gently push it away as if it were a cloud in the sky. Remember that as you continue to think of thoughts that might flood your mind, simply let them pass, not giving them any attention at all. The only thing you should be focusing on now is being as relaxed as possible.

Look in front of you as you close your eyes. Keep your eyes straight forward, and imagine nothing but blackness. Don't drift away into an imagery, or a fantasy. Simply continue to keep your eyes closed. Look ahead of you now into the darkness that is behind your eyelids.

Nothing is in front of you. The only thing that you need to focus on now is being as calm and relaxed as possible. In front of you, you see a little bright light. It is nothing more than the size of a penny. You continue to see it grow and grow.

It gets bigger and bigger, until you see that there is a path in front of you. In your mind, you take a step forward. It is a nature walk. This path is going to take you through the forest.

You are completely at peace, calm, and centered, looking at nothing but what is in front of you. The sidewalk is gray stone, and you take a step forward. You are now completely relaxed. Nothing occupying your mind, other than the sites that you see around you. On your left is a lush green forest. On your right is a large calm and cool body of water. It is a lake, nothing special about it.

It is like many other lakes that you pass. This one in particular is sticking out to you now, because you are more and more relaxed. Now that you have no stress to focus on, you can look ahead of you and see everything that is beautiful about this area. You continue to walk forward, more and more trees emerging each step that you take. On the right, where rocks lines the coast, green leaves stick out through these rocks with large bushes also appearing every once in a while. There are some sticks and other stones lying at the surface of the water with waves splashing against them over and over again.

You continue to walk forward looking at the vast blue on your right. You see a path emerge on the left; you decide to follow it and the sidewalk is now gone. There's nothing but dirt. You take a step forward and you can still see the blue on your right side. You are simply now further and further away from it than you were before. You continue on this path and beneath your feet, you see a log. The log must have fallen recently in a storm. You step over it, ignoring that's even there.

There's nothing in particular about this log that is keeping you down. You simply step over it and continue to move on the path that gets higher and higher and you can see more and more of the blue water next to you. Behind the water is a large mountain covered in lush green. All around you is green, blue, and brown. It is nature, it is the earth, you are connected to it.

You see the blue beneath you. But you continue to step forward on the path. Nothing is getting in your way. You can hear the cicadas, the bees, and other bugs flying around in the woods, but none of this scares you. There's nothing that you have to worry about now. You are simply enjoying all the wonderful sights around you.

You are further and further from the water now elevated several feet above. There's a few more trees and the lush green on your right is getting greater.

Every once in a while, as you keep moving forward, you occasionally notice more branches, trees, and bushes. You notice how nature changes itself without any help. Trees fall but then a new one grows in its place. Flowers bloom. Bees pollinate, and they continue to grow greater and greater. Water is the source of so much of this. Water is where animals and nature connect. Different animals approach the water to drink from it. Birds fly over-top and land in the bushes.

It is a gorgeous site that is keeping you extremely relaxed. You could certainly find something to be afraid of. Maybe the height, the bugs, or even a snake. None of this matters now, however. You only care about being as relaxed as possible. You get to a point where there's a large tree hanging over the trail.

It casts a shadow and gives you a moment to appreciate the darkness; even when the sun is absent this beauty still exists. It even transformed throughout the day as well. Always looking a little bit different.

Throughout all of the green, wild flowers emerge.

It's not like the strict landscaping that you see it in some people's houses. It is nature creating its own beautiful patterns. There are some blue flowers here and some white flowers there.

Sometimes the flowers cross over the path connected only by their color. There are yellow little dots all throughout, some long purple strands, and even a few red flowers. There is no order to this, they simply grow where they had been planted.

Even though it might not have been planned out, they're still so beautiful. Now, a butterfly comes and passes over the path. It continues to fly around you and you appreciate its unique beauty. This used to be something that looked like a little worm, but it is now a beautiful butterfly. You are not afraid of it. You're not afraid of any of these little critters or gorgeous little parts of nature.

You go left a little bit more.

You see another path that takes you deeper into the forest. You're not going to go up to the water anymore. You want to get deeper and deeper into nature. You see birds, leaves, trees, and other gorgeous things above you and swallowing you as if you were becoming part of it yourself. It helps make you completely at peace. There is nothing around you, which scares you in this moment. You are on your own, and that is, OK. You feel completely relaxed and at ease when you are surrounded by greenery. Nothing could ever cause you stress.

When there is so much beauty around you to appreciate, how could you ever have worries over things that are so small? These plants don't have worries. These flowers aren't afraid. You continue, placing one foot in front of the other.

Notice your breath again now. With each step you take in a new breath. Breathe in for one, two, three, four, and five. Breathe out for five, four, three, two, and one.

You are completely at ease. You are entirely relaxed, nothing around you can cause you fear or anxiety. You go deeper and deeper into the forest. There is nothing but trees and wildflowers now. They all stand so tall, pointed towards the sun. The cycle of life is overwhelming. It radiates through your body, and you are reminded of who you truly are. You are not defined by the things that cause you stress. You do not have to worry about what you cannot control. There will always be so many surprises in life, and this does not scare you. It empowers you. There are so many uncertainties that we might run into, but none of this causes you fear, it makes you feel good. It makes you feel strong, it makes you feel brave. You are part of nature, you work with it. You are one with your surroundings.

Breathe in again for five, four, three, two, one, and out for one, two, three, four, and five. Feel as the nature that surrounds you becomes a part of who you are. Each breath that you take is one which fills you with happiness, peace, and serenity. The air you breath sends oxygen all throughout your body, becoming a part of the cycle of your system. You absorb everything around you through the air that you are breathing.

You see nothing around you now but the trees. The water is out of sight, you continue to walk deeper and deeper into the woods. You are entirely at peace, nothing around you that reminds you of what you experienced before is causing you any stress or anxiety now. You are completely and entirely free from the things that used to scare you.

It can be hard to know how to heal ourselves and to reduce our stress when your brain is so stressed out. How could you even possibly manage to think of a way to lift yourself up from this challenging mood? Now, you know, when you are stressed, you can come back to this for those purposes. Each step you take is one dedicated to being more calm. You continue to walk deeper into the woods and ahead of you, you notice a river.

It is a calm stream, but you can still hear the water running. You think about the water that you had just seen, and you realize it must lead to a waterfall.

Maybe one day you'll visit that waterfall. But for now, you choose to step towards the stream and watch as the water passes on the surface of the stream. There are leaves floating towards the waterfall. You can't see the endpoint, but you know where they're going and what their destination is.

You simply watch the leaves pass gently through the stream and away from you.

These leaves can represent your thoughts. Your thoughts can flow gently towards you, and you can choose to stop them. You could choose to stand in front of these leaves and pick them up. If you were submerged yourself in the water, the leaves would stick to you, the same way your beliefs do.

You could change the direction that they move in, but you don't have to do that. You can simply notice the leaves and let them continue on in their journey. Do this with your thoughts as your thoughts trickle in. Just leave them be, let them pass through your mind, and focus your attention on something new. Maybe you'll find that one special leaf that you decide to pick out and choose to keep. That is okay, but you can't do that with every leaf. You have to make it special.

You continue to walk along the stream. Noticing all the different shapes of the little rocks that lay at the bottom.

Every once in a while, you'll see a little fish dart away. Does this fish know where it is? Why does this fish wrongly swim against the current?

Does this fish know what's waiting for it if it follows the current?

What would happen if it did choose to just swim and turn around?

These thoughts simply pass through your mind, but you don't attach an emotion to them. You don't need to feel stressed or scared in this moment, you are perfectly fine. Continue on.

You step further down the stream and you notice the turtle submerging itself into the water. There's a little frog as well hopping around. They enjoy nature, but do they appreciate it the same way you do?

These questions, they don't need answers, but it helps to think about them. It can be a distraction from your stressors. You look up and see a deer. You freeze knowing that if you make any sudden movement, the deer will run away. The deer is not relaxed.

It is always on high alert for anything dangerous that might surround it. The deer does not understand that it doesn't have to live like this. You crouch down letting it know that you are not going to harm it. You look ahead and the deer dips its neck low sticking its tongue out into the cool fresh water. It takes a few sips feeling hydrated and refreshed. You appreciate that this deer is now trusting of you.

It looks back at you before it walks away into the forest. The deer is just like you.

You don't have to be so afraid thinking there is a threat standing across the stream. Sometimes, it could be something that could help you instead.

This fills you with peace. You turn around and decide that it is now time to head back home. You haven't completed the path but you don't have to. It's okay to just enjoy a little bit at a time. Not everything has to be done to completion. You start to walk back, but now you notice all these things so differently. The sun is starting to set, so it's getting darker and darker. More animals are hiding as others emerge. You can hear the sound of crickets as they replace the buzz of cicadas. You hear frogs start to emerge from their daily slumbers to catch any flies or mosquitoes that are going to be out tonight.

What was on one side before is now on the other side as you walk back down the path. You can start to see the water again, the cool blue. There are a few people splashing around and taking a relaxing dip in the distance.

You pay no mind to them, they are having their own fun. You are focused on yourself. You're getting closer and closer now to the beginning of the path, you feel more and more relaxed, you are at peace with yourself and the world in which you live in. There is nothing that scares you. You don't have to be afraid or fearful, nothing's going to harm you. You're more relaxed now than you could ever imagine that you would be. You are leaving this forest, a new person. This walk has changed you. You are now letting go of all the stress and tension that you have been carrying around. There is no need to hold onto stressful thoughts.

You leave all that behind, in nature. It is going to become one with its surroundings. Now, you can see the end of the path, and it is almost night.

Slowly bring yourself back to where you are in the present moment. Feel your breath go in and out. Breathe in for one, two, three, four, and five and out for five, four, three, two, and one. Continue to breathe. Your eyes are still closed and heavy. The forest in front of you is now fading to black. Just like the bright light that emerged earlier, this light is now becoming smaller and smaller.

You are back home again, and you can feel your surroundings. You are connected to them, and one with nature. You are not afraid, fearful, stressed, or angry. You are just you.

As we count down from 20, you will slowly fall into sleep or move on to the next meditation.

Twenty, nineteen, eighteen, seventeen, sixteen, fifteen, fourteen, thirteen, twelve, eleven, ten, nine, eight, seven, six, five, four, three, two, one.

Chapter 11 Affirmation

Affirmations are phrases that usually start with "I" and include ideas that we can start to incorporate in our own minds. We often state affirmations to ourselves all day, but it can be hard to notice. They become ingrained in the way we think, and unfortunately, they are often negative affirmations.

These positive affirmations will make it easier to have healthier sleeping habits in your life. The more you can include these in your vocabulary, the easier it will become to see better sleep habits forming in your life.

Sleep Affirmations

To best practice using affirmations, say them to yourself as often as possible, especially when you are having negative thoughts. Even if you don't fully believe them at first, they will help you to eventually turn around your patterns of thinking.

Write them down and include notes throughout your house with the affirmations stated on them. Set alarms with these affirmations to help you remember to consistently include these patterns of thoughts into the way that you think. Below is a list of positive affirmations you can use to help improve your sleep.

Healthy Sleep Habits Affirmations

1. I am always looking for ways to improve my health.
2. I choose to incorporate habits in my life that will make everything else better as well.
3. I sleep when I am tired.
4. I wake up when I have had enough sleep.
5. I don't stare at my phone as I fall asleep.
6. I make sure to feel relaxed before going to bed.
7. When I have had enough sleep, everything else in my life will be better.
8. I have better focus when I am well-rested.
9. I have a better memory when I've had enough sleep.
10. It feels good to get the right amount of sleep and to take care of myself.
11. I feel better every day with each healthy habit I choose to include in my life.
12. I deserve to feel well-rested.

13. Getting the right amount of sleep is natural for me.

14. It is naturally healthy to ensure that I am centered on getting the best sleep possible.

15. I am always looking for ways to improve my sleep.

16. I do not allow myself to make bad decisions for my health when I know better.

17. I go to bed at the right time even if there is a distraction that keeps me up.

18. I make sure that I do not do anything that will prevent me from getting the right amount of sleep.

19. I allow myself to wind down before actually going to sleep.

20. My mind, body, and soul feel better when I have had the right amount of sleep.

Relaxing Affirmations

1. I feel more and more relaxed as I attempt to get the right amount of sleep.

2. I feel the relaxation throughout my mind.

3. I feel relaxed in every part of my body.

4. I am filled with peace.

5. I pour out serenity to those around me.

6. I am focused on becoming calmer and calmer.

7. I am not afraid of anything that might come my way.

8. I do not dwell on things that have already happened.

9. I release myself from the stress that I have already felt.

10. I do not restrict myself with fear over things that might be out of my control.

11. I know what is in and out of my control.

12. I fall asleep fast so that I can get the most amount of rest possible.

13. I do not fear stress; I know how to experience it at a healthy level.

14. I am excited about what tomorrow holds.

15. I do not fear the challenges I face.

16. I let the past stay in the past and do not let it drive my future.

17. I am present in this moment and focused on relaxing.

18. I relax throughout the day so that I can sleep better at night.

19. I sleep most peacefully when I release myself from my anxieties.

20. Peace and serenity are my normal states of being.

Deep Sleep Affirmations

1. I do not allow distractions that will keep me up all night.

2. I feel completely relaxed in my bed.

3. I surround myself with peace before I go to bed.

4. I fall asleep fast and make sure that I stay that way throughout the night.

5. I feel safe as I sleep, which helps me get a deeper rest.

6. I am able to fall back asleep even if I wake up at night.

7. I do not allow past restless nights to define how I will be sleeping now.

8. I make sure that everything around me promotes comfort so that I can stay focused on right now.

9. Sleep is a requirement for my health.

10. I am deserving of a deep and restful night's sleep.

11. I cut out habits that keep me from getting a deep sleep.

12. I separate myself from electronics in order to promote better sleep.

13. I focus on sleeping the moment that I lay down for bed.

14. I always focus on my health so that I can get a deeper sleep.

15. I clear my mind before bed so that I focus on nothing other than drifting away.

16. I feel refreshed after making decisions for better relaxation.

17. I manage my sleep in the healthiest ways possible.

18. Deep sleep gives me a deeper ability to process my thoughts.

19. Stress does not consume me.

20. I am always focused on healthy sleeping.

Chapter 12   Understanding Hypnosis - History, Benefits, and Uses

All of us are familiar with the rather clichéd and stereotypical line, "You are slowly falling asleep" that is connected with hypnotism, right? In fact, this line leads us to believe that hypnosis is something 'bad' and a hypnotist can control us completely during a hypnotic state. Similarly, you may have seen stage hypnosis, when the phenomenon is said to be 'magical.'

However, in truth, like meditation, hypnosis is a useful self-development tool to live life more meaningfully and happily than before. Hypnosis can be seen as a form of meditation to achieve a specific goal. Meditation and hypnosis are similar concepts in the fact that both are excellent tools to achieve a state of deep relaxation and concentration.

So, what is hypnosis? It is a mental state where you achieve supremely focused concentration, heightened suggestibility, and reduced peripheral awareness. Hypnosis is a genuine psychological phenomenon that has multiple therapeutic uses in clinical practice. The process of hypnotism typically includes three distinct steps, namely:

- *Hypnotic Induction* - This is the process that is used to achieve hypnosis. Ideally, the person undergoing hypnosis is made to sit comfortably in a chair or made to lie down on a couch or bed with eyes closed. Controlled breathing techniques can also be used to enhance the feeling of comfort. Then, a memorized script, tape recording, or a live hypnotherapist is used in the process of hypnotic induction.

- *Hypnotic State* - This state is achieved after hypnotic induction. The hypnotic state represents a calm, focused state of mind with heightened awareness. In this state, the person in a hypnotic state feels physically and mentally relaxed.

- *Hypnotic Suggestion* - When the person reaches the hypnotic state, he or she is ready to receive hypnotic suggestions, created to replace automatic thoughts in the subconscious mind. Suggestions can be formulated in different ways; the traditional methods involve suggestions given as direct commands to the subconscious mind. In Ericksonian hypnosis, metaphors are used to make suggestions. In the neuro-linguistic programming method, suggestions mimic the patient's thought patterns.

Trained experts employ a multitude of techniques to induce a hypnotic state in people. The power of suggestion is one of the primary reasons why hypnosis is used for relaxation, reduction of pain, and to bring about positive behavioral changes.

Hypnosis is also referred to as a hypnotic suggestion or hypnotherapy. Hypnotherapists combine soothing verbal repetitions and mental imagery to get patients into a trance-like state. When patients are totally and completely relaxed, therapists use suggestive messages to bring about positive transformations in the mind of the person under hypnosis.

Interestingly, research has proved that not all human beings are equally hypnotizable. Some people appear to be more open to suggestions and hypnotherapy than others. The 'hypnotizability' trait differs from person to person. Brain imaging techniques reveal that patterns in brain connectivity differ in people who are responsive to hypnotherapy and those who are not.

Before we move on to understand more about hypnosis, it might make sense to know the differences between the various terms used in this field.

- *Hypnosis* - Also referred to as the hypnotic state, hypnosis is the highly focused and relaxed state of mind that is reached after being hypnotized.

- *Hypnotism* - The process of hypnotic induction used to achieve the hypnotic state is called hypnotism.

- *Hypnotherapy* - This term refers to the use of hypnosis and hypnotism as a therapeutic tool. Hypnotherapists are trained and qualified professionals who help people to achieve hypnosis-powered self-development goals.

The Truth about Hypnosis

For a long time, hypnosis was considered to be one of the most controversial and misunderstood methods of psychological therapy. Misconceptions and myths surrounding hypnotherapy are mostly based on hypnotism produced by stage artists and magicians, which is nothing but a theatrical performance and has nothing in common with hypnosis being used as psychological therapy.

In a hypnotic state, people appear to be more open to suggestions than in their normal state. Positive suggestions given to people during hypnosis are called "post-hypnotic suggestions." They do not take effect until the person has emerged from the hypnotic state.

The suggestions given to people, when they are in the hypnotic state, play a crucial role in the entire process of hypnotherapy. Direct suggestions to bring about positive changes are typically not responded to by people in the normal psychological state of mind. However, during hypnosis, it seems that suggestions make a 'backdoor' entry into the consciousness of the affected person. This place is believed to be the root of important psychological or behavioral changes.

Another important myth to be dismissed is that people under hypnosis are not in control of themselves. Nothing can be further from the truth. Hypnotized people are completely in control of themselves and will not act or do anything objectionable or harmful to themselves or others.

For a person to undergo hypnotherapy for positive results, he or she must participate in the process voluntarily and must have the ability to be hypnotized. In fact, highly hypnotizable people do not always benefit from hypnotherapy.

Moreover, hypnotherapy is not a one-session treatment where lasting changes can be expected. People typically have to undergo a series of procedures to reinforce constructive suggestions repeatedly for positive changes to take place. The most common use of hypnotherapy is to break bad habits, recalling and acknowledging past forgotten memories, overcoming stress, anxiety, and insomnia, and for managing pain.

History of Hypnosis

While stage hypnosis and its related 'magical' effects are relatively new, the idea of hypnosis has been in use in the field of Western psychology for thousands of centuries. Eastern religions like Hinduism have self-hypnosis as part of their religious rituals. In the 11th century, Avicenna, a famed physician from Persia, is credited with documenting the concept of hypnotism.

One of the earliest forms of using hypnosis as a distinct therapy in the field of psychology is given to Franz Anton Mesmer, an 18th-century healer. Mesmer was a strong believer in astrological principles and opined that heavenly bodies have a direct influence on the physical, emotional, and mental health of human beings.

Initially, Mesmer used magnets in grand, theatrical ways resulting in expected spasmodic muscular contractions, which, in turn, frequently resulting in curing of illnesses. Mesmer used rationalistic terms like magnetism and gravitation for his healing methods. He said that these healing methods can influence the subtle fluids within the human body. His methods and subsequent subsets established by others are collectively referred to as Mesmerism.

Even though Mesmer and his methods were discredited, later on, he was able to convince his followers that they can channelize their 'animal magnetism' to cure and alleviate the symptoms of their illnesses and ailments.

The earliest distinction between Mesmer's kind of 'mesmerism' and modern hypnotherapy was made by Dr. James Braid, a Manchester surgeon who coined the term 'hypnosis' in 1843. The term has its roots in the name of the Greek God of Sleep Hypnos because most forms of mesmerism involved a sleep-like status for the patient. Braid proposed that the reason for Mesmer's methods having some effect on followers was the power of suggestion.

Braid worked with hypnotherapy, and in his early studies, he thought that hypnosis could result in a unique condition of the nervous system that could be suitable for suggestion-based cures. However, further studies made him reject his own theory, and he emphasized the importance of "mental factors" playing a role in hypnotherapy.

However, the neural connection was not entirely dismissed. Ivan Pavlov, an important figure who contributed immensely to the field of psychology, worked on the neural inhibition theory as part of his research on the physiology of sleep. Many of Pavlov's ideas have proven to be fairly accurate in a general sense.

Jean Marie-Charcot was a French neurologist who started using hypnosis as a therapy to cure a disorder highly prevalent during her time, namely hysteria (which, in Greek, which translates to "wandering uterus"). Sigmund Freud studied this concept with Charcot. However, as he was not a very good hypnotist, he used this theory of reaching the subconscious mind of patients through free association.

Modern-day hypnotherapy was founded in the early 20th century by members of a society called "Nancy School of Hypnosis." The elaborate theories on hypnotic therapy proposed by the founding members of this group replaced many of the older ideas, including the neural connections as well as Braid's early theories based on magnetism and gravitation.

Freud also believed in the theories of the Nancy School, believing that people generally tend to repress painful and traumatic memories. He believed that hypnotherapy could help such people come to terms with these traumatic memories and cure mental and psychological problems rooted in the repressed and forgotten memories.

Other important psychologists who contributed to the field of hypnotherapy included Clark Hull (his 1933 discussion based on his research is still used by modern therapists and is considered a classic), Milton Erickson (whose name is most closely connected to clinical hypnosis today), and Jay Hayley (who developed the MRI Interactional Model of therapy). Neuro-Linguistic Programming (NLP) is one of the most popular forms of hypnotherapy used by therapists across the world today.

The research on hypnotherapy continues, with people from all over the world reaping the benefits.

Common Misconceptions about Hypnosis

Hypnotists cannot make you do anything against your will. No, they cannot make you cluck like a hen or any such ridiculous thing. Hypnosis is not a tool to control the mind. Instead, it is very similar to meditation and allows you to enter into a state of deep relaxation and concentration. The person undergoing hypnosis is in complete control of himself or herself. Here are some common misconceptions about hypnosis for your reference and better understanding:

You are unconscious or asleep - The deep state of relaxation and concentration is frequently mistaken for a state of unconsciousness or deep sleep. While the origin of the word is rooted in Hypnos, the Greek God of Sleep, in reality, you don't go to sleep. Under the influence of hypnosis, you are fully awake and are acutely aware of your surroundings and what is happening to you.

You lose control - This idea is a total myth. The person under hypnotic induction experiences a heightened level of concentration and focus. All distractions are tuned out, and he or she achieve total relaxation. The person under hypnosis can open his or her eyes at any time and is in complete control.

Hypnosis is a magic pill - Hypnosis does not promise to cure anything and everything. You should have a deep desire to make a positive difference in your life, and hypnotherapy is a tool that will help you achieve your desire. However, you have to work at it. Hypnosis is not a magic pill.

You can get stuck in a hypnotic state - Many movies depict scenes where the villain hypnotizes someone, and this person can never wake up at all because he or she remains hypnotized forever! This scene is only for fictional movies and does not happen in reality. In real life hypnosis sessions, you can open your eyes and come back to your surroundings anytime you want.

How Does Hypnotherapy Work?

To understand how hypnosis works, you must know how your subconscious (or unconscious) mind works. The subconscious mind controls nearly all of our thoughts and thinking processes. A significant portion of our thoughts originates automatically through the unconscious mind. This is the place where good and bad habits get stuck driven by our repeated and reinforced actions. All our fears, doubts, and worries are also seated in the unconscious mind.

For example, a negative experience could have resulted in the development of fear of flying. Regardless of the intensity of the experience, your emotional reactions could have been so strong that your unconscious mind associates flying as being a life-threatening risk. This kind of phobia is also stored in the subconscious mind.

In simple terms, hypnosis changes the way we feel, perceive, think, sense, and act, while following someone else's suggestions. Hypnotic suggestions are most effective when you suspend your conscious control over your thoughts and behaviors. Of course, this calls for a serious level of commitment? After all, why would anyone hand over control of his or her mind to someone else?

The thing is that a good and well-trained hypnotherapist can convince you that you are in good and trustworthy hands even while you are only in a partially hypnotic state. Of course, all qualified therapists are trained to teach people to believe in their expertise and assure their clients that no harm will befall them. The fact that the most important element of hypnotherapy is suggestion makes it vital that the therapist is in control of the therapy session so that the client finds it easy to hand over control of his or her mental cognition.

The second vital element of hypnosis is the "focus of attention." Most hypnotists will tell their clients that the process is nothing more than focusing attention. Can you recall the experience of watching a movie that you were thoroughly engrossed in? Reading a book that you couldn't put down? Well, both could easily qualify as a hypnotic session. You are, effectively, so engrossed in the movie or the book that you forget everything else going on around you.

The element referred to as the "focus of attention" in hypnotherapy works on similar lines. You are so focused on the therapist's voice that your own thoughts are turned off. Now it becomes easy for the therapist to suggest and implant his or her own words, depending on the expected outcome of the therapy.

It is important to remember that all external noise cannot be really be quietened down in a hypnotherapy session, especially in a group session. In such situations, therapists use something called a 'paradoxical' statement, which helps to keep these disturbing external noises out of your focus.

The third vital element of hypnosis is relaxation, one of the primary reasons for people to turn to hypnotherapy. When the therapist secures your focus on attention, he or she can take you through a standard series of relaxation exercises. Typically, the hypnotherapist will ask you to slowly unwind and untwist the knots and tensions of your muscles, starting from the feet upward, similar to a body-scan meditation therapy.

Hypnotherapy is excellent for relaxation. Your eyes are closed, and you are asked to unwind completely, allowing yourself to slip down into the couch. The voice of the hypnotherapist helps you to prevent your own thoughts getting in the way of relaxation and rest.

The fourth element of hypnotherapy is imagery. The hypnotherapist helps you to imagine scenes facilitating the focus of attention. For example, the therapist asks you to imagine that you are slowly and steadily heading down a flight of stairs or in an elevator or even an escalator. A countdown is given as you begin your journey downward, and by the time you reach the bottom, you are in a hypnotic trance, totally focused on the voice of the therapist.

At the end of the session, the therapist again uses the imagery in the reverse order. For example, he or she will tell you to imagine you are walking steadily and slowly walking up a flight of stairs, or in an escalator or elevator. Here too, the countdown begins, and you get out of your hypnotic trance as you get closer to the top.

So, now you may pose the question "How does your hypnotherapist help you when you are in a 'trance' or 'asleep?'" The mystery of hypnotism begins in this state, right? How can you obey your therapist and take his or her suggestions if you are asleep? How can you hear what the therapist is telling you when you are 'sleeping?' Moreover, if it was only to get an hour's sleep, why would people spend money to see a therapist?

Therefore, it can be concluded that hypnotism does involve an altered state of consciousness during which we retain some conscious awareness, which helps us remember what happened after the hypnotic session. So, the question is not "How does hypnosis work?' but "Why does it work?"

Nicolas Spanos, a Canadian psychologist of the 20th century, explained the working of hypnotism, which is accepted even today. Spanos believed that hypnosis does not change the mental state of people. It facilitates the enactment of social roles played by the patient and hypnotist through which positive suggestions are implanted in the mind of the patient. The patient goes for treatment to the hypnotherapist, expecting to be hypnotized. Therefore, even though the patient appears to be sleeping, he or she can hear everything and follow the instructions of the hypnotist because he is playing the role of a patient.

Milton Erickson came up with another explanation for why hypnotism works. His method of hypnotism was not based on relaxation but the use of special language and communication. He would repeat the same idea multiple times to his client, either using the same words or different words and phrases until the patient literally falls asleep, akin to a student falling asleep in a boring lecture.

He also used story-telling metaphors to bring on the hypnotic trance likening the tale to the patient's state of mind and then implanting images of success into his or her mind. Both Spanos and Erickson contributed significantly to our understanding of how and why hypnosis works for human beings.

Chapter 13   The First Steps to Ending the Insomnia Struggle

Insomnia, in medical terms, is one of the massive diseases worldwide. Insomnia statistics are growing every day. Today, about 29% of men, 37% of women, 25% of children, and 75% of pregnant women suffer from this disease. Insomnia is expressed in disturbed sleep. Patients are far from always seriously taking insomnia and simply let their treatment "go" on its own. This attitude leads to unpleasant and dangerous consequences in the form of the transition of the disease into a chronic form, neurological disorders, pathologies of internal organs, and mental disorders. Not everyone can cope with insomnia on their own, and in most cases, to get a good result, the help of a medical specialist is needed.

Insomnia, in short, is a widespread phenomenon that is a violation of the quality and quantity of sleep, adversely affecting human daily activities.

Occasionally, it happens in each of us. But when a person spends night after night without sleep - this is a completely different matter. Insomnia is almost always a reflection of other disorders. It testifies either to failures in the physical state, or to emotional experiences.

Often, chronic diseases accompanied by pain (say, arthritis) do not give an opportunity to close your eyes for a moment. After a quarrel with your soul mate, you can also spend the night without sleep. And the troubles at work can turn into the fact that a person tosses and turns under the covers until morning.

In addition, sometimes, there are enough changes in the usual rhythm of life to cause sleep disturbances. For example, due to work on the night shift or because of different time zones.

According to experts, insomnia often begins with a few nights when it is not possible to fall asleep, say, after an injury or emotional upheaval. After such nights, snacking during the day can become a habit, and at night, unsuccessful attempts to fall asleep. A person begins to watch television programs while lying in bed or to visit the refrigerator in the middle of the night. Before he has time to realize what is happening to him, new habits acquire a systematic character. Such disorders are known as habitual insomnia.

All the efforts made by most people to normalize sleep, in reality, only worsen it. The root causes disappear, and insomnia, sadly, remains. Bad habits are fixed that don't allow a person to fall asleep: people begin to constantly look at their watches; as the night closes in, they become anxious.

The sleep rhythm of people suffering from chronic insomnia is so unsettled that they resemble one frantically dancing to the measured melody of an old waltz. What are the signs of chronic insomnia?

- You have difficulty falling asleep almost every evening for several weeks.

- You are overwhelmed with fear of going to bed because you doubt whether you can fall asleep.

- You feel very tired during the day and cannot concentrate in order to work normally.

- You resort to alcohol or medication in order to fall asleep.

Positive Thinking

It is necessary to have a positive attitude not only to oneself but also to life. No doctor can give us health if we ourselves do not take an active part in the process of our own healing. Man must enjoy life. I want to teach you how to use positive thinking to defeat your illnesses.

The point of power is here and now - in our head. And it doesn't matter how long ago negative thoughts began to prevail in us, relations with others deteriorated, finances ran out, self-hatred appeared, and illness came. It's never too late to start changing. Until now, our life and our experience have been created by the thoughts that we kept in mind, as well as those words that we constantly used. Nevertheless, such thinking now belongs to the past; we have already overcome this line. What our tomorrow, the day after tomorrow, the next week, month, year, etc., depends on our current, momentary thoughts and words. The point of application of force is always in the current moment.

Now - this is when we begin to change our lives. What a liberating thought! We can begin to part with the old nonsense. Right now. Even the smallest initial step can be decisive. Here are the first steps to getting rid of insomnia, at whatever stage it might be.

Autogenic Training

The basic principles of autogenic training were developed by the German neuropathologist Johannes Heinrich Schultz at the beginning of the 19th century. Having published several articles in special journals, in 1932, he presented to the medical community, his method described in the monograph "Autogenic training - concentrated self-relaxation."

According to Schultz, auto-training is more suitable for people of an intellectual type, who also have the necessary perseverance. However, in this book, I aim to familiarize you with simple natural techniques that will be useful for improving your well-being. In this case, self-help is understood as a conscious decision to join in the simplified exercises outlined here.

A characteristic feature of autogenous training is the gradual mastery of certain exercises in order to learn how to control the work of internal organs and achieve mental and physical relaxation.

Along with other factors, two fundamental observations served as the impetus for creating an autogenic training. The first is the establishment by Oskar Vogt of the fact that a person who is able to bring himself into a hypnotic state can achieve "deep peace and complete rest" in this way. In this sense, autogenic training is also a way of switching the body from an intense working state to a state of rest. One of the goals of the exercises is to make this transition as inconspicuous and fleeting as possible - "in no time."

In the process of self-hypnosis, a change of state occurs in a strictly defined, unchanging sequence, namely:

1. The necessary posture is taken, and relaxation sets in.
2. The eyes are closed.
3. There is a feeling of general reassurance.
4. A feeling of heaviness appears.
5. There is a pleasant sensation of a feeling of warmth spreading throughout the body.

Exercises

As outlined, we shall start the following exercises:

1. Taking the right pose.
2. The closure of the eyelids.
3. Achieving a sense of comfort.
4. Development of a feeling of heaviness.
5. Nap.

It must be remembered that clothing must be comfortable, not interfering with concentrated self-relaxation. The collar must be unfastened, a tie, a belt, tight shoes to relax or remove.

Pose

For classes, you need to choose a position so that "whenever possible, eliminate any mechanical stress." The body should be completely relaxed and be in it without the use of muscular effort. For auto-training, the following three poses are recommended.

1. "Reclining": This position is best taken in a chair deep enough, with a high back, so that the lower back is located comfortably, and it would be possible to conveniently tilt your head. The armrests should be at such a height that you can put slightly bent elbows on them.

2. "Sitting": An ordinary chair of the appropriate height with a not too soft seat is suitable for this pose. The center of gravity falls on the pelvis or ischium. At the same time, the loin is straightened, and the upper body is slightly bent and resembles the bent back of a cat. The head is relaxed and lowered perpendicular to the pelvis, not the femur. Otherwise, the stomach will be squeezed. The legs are placed at shoulder level, hands are resting on the knees without stopping, and the hands hang freely between the hips: like a coachman who relaxed, weakened the reins, and his horses rave by themselves. If the wrists are completely relaxed, then this is a sure sign that the body position is chosen correctly.

The pose is widely used in group exercises.

3. "Lying": A comfortable, free posture is taken, with the head resting on a pillow. The legs are extended; you can't cross your legs. The feet are slightly outward, which helps to relieve muscle tension. The arms are extended along the torso with palms down and slightly bent at the elbows.

Eyelid Closure

Eyes are closed only after the correct relaxed posture has been adopted. Along with other factors, the meaning of closing the eyelids is to turn off optical irritation, so that during the next exercise - achieving calm - you can use projection in the dark if necessary.

In this case, you should not make any special, deliberate movements of the eyeball, such as looking up and inside. It is only a matter of simply closing the eyes.

Reaching Calm

Only now is the time to move on to "general tuning formulas" (according to Schulz). "Configuring" is carried out using the phrase: "I am completely calm." This phrase is necessary while maintaining the relaxation of the body with eyes closed, to "create" in your imagination as distinctly as possible. It turns out that the phrase can occur in the imagination in various forms, depending on the personality characteristics of the person.

Imagination can be "optical" when a person sees this phrase as if written "in the dark space of the eye" (projection in the dark), or acoustic, in which it is perceived in the form of sound, often with different and variable stresses. If the graphic or sound form has a distinct rhythm, then the person, at least partially, belongs to the artistic type. Representatives of a purely artistic type can recreate this phrase in the form of an image, rhythm, pulsation, etc. And finally, there is a sharply expressed mental type of people, "whose form of imagination does not rely upon or is only limited to rely on sensually-shaped phenomena."

Schulz strongly emphasizes that the phrase mentioned is solely intended to bring into a state of drowsiness and in no case, should be taken as a "calming exercise."

The development of a feeling of heaviness

As already mentioned, the phrase "I am completely calm" is not an exercise for training. It serves only to tune your own "I."

The center of consciousness is intended for thought, which is currently being inspired. If the exercise is successful, then in the corresponding arm, lying calmly, a sensation of muscle heaviness really appears. But an attempt (out of curiosity or for control) to raise this hand leads to the exact opposite effect - the hand seems quite light. The feeling of heaviness arises in this case due to relaxation.

When the exercise is successful, the muscles are completely relaxed and supple.

Exit from the Nap State

The first lesson in an autogenic training course ends with the development of a sensation of muscle heaviness. If, after finishing this exercise, you try to get up immediately, this can lead to various unpleasant consequences. Therefore, it is very important to correctly get out of the state. It must be remembered that you are actually in a state of self-hypnosis, although your consciousness is not turned off. The physical part of your "I" is also in a more or less deep hypnotic state, like a hypnotized body.

The exit from autogenic immersion is carried out in three stages:

1. It is necessary several times to bend sharply and unbend the arm, heavy as a result of self-hypnosis.
2. Take a deep, full breath.
3. And only then open your eyes.

The sequence of action when exiting a nap must be observed very accurately and strictly. In no case should you treat it carelessly? It is an integral part of the auto-training process and is as important as the previous steps. With this sequence, a person returns to a normal awake state.

After the correct exit from a nap, the first lesson ends. In exactly two weeks, according to Schultz, one can achieve a "satisfactory generalization" of good feelings. Only after this can we move on to the next step - developing a sensation of a feeling of warmth.

Conclusion

No more nights wasted in the isolation of insomnia. No more nights spent frustrated that you are awake at three in the morning. No more nights that you are forfeiting to insomnia. No more mornings ruined by stress, anxiety, and depression. Finally, you have found the key to waking up relaxed and refreshed, fully restored after a good night's sleep. Hypnosis is the solution to your insomnia.

So many other solutions have come up short. However, now you have your secret to achieving sleep. The hypnosis sessions can be used as often as you need. They are a tool for you to sleep your way to the life you want to lead: a life of happiness and relaxation. You have explored the benefits of sleep hypnosis and its potential as a solution to insomnia. You have experienced its effectiveness for yourself with these four highly-successful guided meditations. You are ready to improve your quality of life by enhancing your quality of sleep. Sleep well.

CPSIA information can be obtained
at www.ICGtesting.com
Printed in the USA
LVHW101135280221
678894LV00045B/1031